AF323405

CANCER, DIAGNOSTICS, and CHEMOTHERAPY

A REFERENCE MANUAL

CYNTHIA C. CHERNECKY, MN, PhC, RN

CANCER, DIAGNOSTICS, and CHEMOTHERAPY

A REFERENCE MANUAL

Cynthia C. Chernecky, MN, PhC, RN

Clinical Nurse Specialist in Oncology
St. Joseph's Hospital
Atlanta, Georgia

W.B. SAUNDERS COMPANY
A Division of Harcourt Brace & Company

Philadelphia   London   Toronto   Montreal   Sydney   Tokyo

W.B. SAUNDERS COMPANY
A Division of
Harcourt Brace & Company

The Curtis Center
Independence Square West
Philadelphia, PA 19106

Editor: Michael J. Brown
Designer: Patti Maddaloni
Production Manager: Peter Faber
Manuscript Editor: Gina Scala

Cancer, Diagnostics, and Chemotherapy: A Reference Manual   ISBN 0-7216-3187-8

Copyright © 1991 by W.B. Saunders Company.

All rights reserved. No part of this publication may be reproduced or transmitted in any form or by any means, electronic or mechanical, including photocopy, recording, or any information storage and retrieval system, without permission in writing from the publisher. Library of Congress catalog card number 91-10446.

Printed in the United States of America.

Last digit is the print number: 9 8 7 6 5 4 3 2

My heartfelt thanks to my mom, Olga, who enriched me with life, love, and the profession of nursing. To my brother Richard who has filled my life with brotherly love and inspired me through his profession, medicine. To my godmother, Helen Prohorik, whose heart and soul as an orthodox Christian have always been an inspiration to me. To Ruth Krech, MSN, RN, whose friendship and hours of brainstorming helped me sustain my motivation. To Julie and Charles Dewey, whose love of family has been of great importance to me. I thank all of you for your special gifts!

Finally, I would like to acknowledge those academic institutions that have been a part of my professional growth: The University of Connecticut, The University of Pittsburgh, Clemson University, and Case Western Reserve University.

Dedication

Preface

This manual is intended to meet two clinical needs: the need for nurses to have a quick reference source, and the need for an easy-to-use, not overwhelming list of side effects with which to educate clients and that clients can keep as a reference for themselves.

This manual has three sections. In Part I, Cancer Profiles, areas of the body where cancer occurs are listed in alphabetical order along with risk factors, signs and symptoms (the most common one flagged with an asterisk), diagnostic tests used most often in evaluating or diagnosing the cancer, generalized survival statistics, and the most common sites of metastases from each specific cancer. These profiles assist professionals in assessment and planning. In Part II, Diagnostic Tests, the diagnostic tests found in Part I are listed in alphabetical order and are defined, and pre-care and post-care are described when significant. In Part III, Chemotherapeutic Agents, each card has two sides: one for the nurse and the other for the client. The nurse's information consists of the drug's names, action, nadir, side effects (including whether the drug is a vesicant and how to treat the extravasation), special conditions about each side effect, and types of cancers against which the drug is known to be effective. The client's information consists of side effects listed in alphabetical order, described in everyday language. An index of cross-referencing for chemotherapeutic drug names follows for easy access.

CC

Pauline M. Baca, RNC
Anna Cate, BSN, RN
Patricia Roush Honas, BSN, RN
Deborah Jay, RN
Laura McKillop, RN
Pat Sasso, RN
Debra Ann Ropelewski-Zanath, BSN, RNC

Special thanks to Pat Franta, MSN, RN,
for her assistance in the early part of this project.

Acknowledgments

PART I · CANCER PROFILES · 2

Bladder · 3

Bone · 4

Brain · 5

Breast · 6

Central Nervous System · 7

Cervix · 8

Colon · 9

Endometrium · 10

Esophagus · 11

Contents

Gallbladder · 12

Head and Neck · 13

Hodgkin's Disease · 14

Kidney · 15

Larynx · 16

Leukemia in Children · 17

Leukemia in Adults · 18

Liver · 19

Lung · 20

Lymphoma, Non-Hodgkin's · 21

Melanoma · 22
Multiple Myeloma · 23
Neuroblastoma · 24
Oral Cavity · 25
Ovary · 26
Pancreas · 27
Prostate · 28
Rectum · 29
Retinoblastoma · 30
Skin, Nonmelanoma Types · 31

Stomach · 32

Testes · 33

Thyroid · 34

Uterus · 35

Vagina · 36

Vulva · 37

Wilms' Tumor · 38

PART II · DIAGNOSTIC TESTS · 40

Acid Phosphatase, Serum · 41

AFP · 41

Amylase, Serum · 41

Barium Esophagogram · 42

BE · 42

Biopsy · 43

Biopsy Using Toluidine Blue 10% Solution · 43

Bone Marrow Aspiration · 43

Bone Scan · 44

Bronchial Washings · 44

Brushings Cytology · 44

Contents

B-Subunit HCG · 44

CBC · 45

CEA · 45

Chest Radiograph · 45

Colonoscopy · 46

Colposcopy · 46

Conizaton · 46

CT Scan · 47

Cystoscopy · 47

Digital Examination · 47

EEG · 48
Endocervical Curettage · 48
Endoscopic Examination · 48
ERCP · 48
Esophagoscopy · 49
Glucose, Blood · 49
Hemogram · 50
History and Physical Examination · 50
Inferior Venacavography · 50
Iron, Serum · 50

IVP · 51
Liver Function Tests · 51
Liver Profile, Serum · 52
Liver Scan · 52
Lower GI Series · 52
Lumbar Puncture · 52
Mammography · 53
Monoclonal Antibodies · 53
MRI · 54
NSE Tumor Marker, Serum · 54

Nuclear Imaging with MIBG · 54

OCA-125 Antigen, Serum · 54

Occult Blood, Stool · 55

Pap Test · 55

PET · 55

Prostate-Specific Antigen · 55

PTC · 56

PTT · 56

Radiograph, Bone · 56

Radiograph, Skeletal · 56

Radiograph, Skull · 57

Rectal Examination · 57

Renal Angiography · 57

Renal Ultrasonography · 57

Sedimentation Rate, Blood · 58

Serum Electrophoresis, M Component · 58

Sigmoidoscopy · 58

SMA-20 · 58

Sputum Cytology · 59

Thyroid Scan · 59

Ultrasound · 59
Upper GI Series · 59
Urinalysis · 60
Urine HVA · 60
Urine VMA · 60
Visual Inspection of Oral Cavity · 60
X-ray · 60

PART III · CHEMOTHERAPEUTIC AGENTS · 62
L-Asparaginase · 64

Contents

Contents

Bleomycin Sulfate · 66

Busulfan · 68

Carboplatin · 70

Carmustine · 72

Chlorambucil · 74

Chlorotrianisene · 76

Cisplatin · 78

Colony-Stimulating Factor · 80

Cyclophosphamide · 82

Cytarabine · 84

Dacarbazine · 86
Dactinomycin · 88
Daunorubicin Hydrochloride · 90
Dexamethasone · 92
Diethylstilbestrol · 94
Doxorubicin Hydrochloride · 96
Estramustine Phosphate Sodium · 98
Estrogens, Conjugated · 100
Etoposide · 102
Floxuridine · 104

Contents

5-Fluorouracil · 106

Fluoxymesterone · 108

Hexamethylmelamine · 110

Hydrocortisone Sodium Succinate · 112

Hydroxyurea · 114

Ifosfamide · 116

Interferon · 118

Interleukin-2 · 120

Leucovorin · 122

Leuprolide Acetate · 124

Lomustine · 126

Mechlorethamine Hydrochloride · 128

Medroxyprogesterone Acetate · 130

Megestrol Acetate · 132

Melphalan · 134

6-Mercaptopurine · 136

Methotrexate · 138

Methylprednisolone Sodium Succinate · 140

Mitomycin C · 142

Mitotane · 144

Contents xxiii

Contents

Mitoxantrone Hydrochloride · 146

Monoclonal Antibodies · 148

Plicamycin · 150

Prednisone · 152

Procarbazine Hydrochloride · 154

Semustine · 156

Streptozotocin · 158

Tamoxifen Citrate · 160

Teniposide · 162

Testosterone · 164

Thioguanine · 166

Thiotepa · 168

Tumor Necrosis Factor · 170

Vinblastine Sulfate · 172

Vincristine Sulfate · 174

Vindesine Sulfate · 176

BIBLIOGRAPHY · 178

INDEX OF CHEMOTHERAPEUTIC AGENTS · 179

CANCER, DIAGNOSTICS, and CHEMOTHERAPY

A REFERENCE MANUAL

PART I

CANCER PROFILES

Cancer	Risk Factors	Signs and Symptoms	Diagnostic Tests	Survival
Bladder Metastasis: kidney, nodes	Age >50 years; white race; male sex; smoking; vitamin A decreased	*Hematuria; dysuria; pyuria; urinary frequency	CT, abdomen; CT, pelvis; cystoscopy; cytology; IVP; urinalysis	70%, 5-year

Cancer	Risk Factors	Signs and Symptoms	Diagnostic Tests	Survival
Bone Metastases: lung, nodes	Age 20–30 years; age 60–70 years; white race	*Pain, deep; pain, agonizing; pain at night	Bone scan; CT scan; monoclonal antibodies; MRI; radiograph, bone	50–80%, 5-year

Cancer	Risk Factors	Signs and Symptoms	Diagnostic Tests	Survival
Brain Metastases: meninges	Age <10 years old; age 55–79 years old; barbiturate use; white race; exposure to high-dose x-rays; lead exposure; male sex; sodium nitrate food consumption; work with chemicals, pesticides, rubber, and oil, and in embalming	*Headache; personality changes; seizures; vomiting	CT, head; EEG; MRI; PET	25%, 2-year

Cancer	Risk Factors	Signs and Symptoms	Diagnostic Tests	Survival
Breast Metastases: bone, brain, liver, lung, meninges, nodes	Family history of breast cancer; female sex; fibrocystic change in breast; high-fat diet; residence in industrialized countries; menstruation prior to age 12 years; menopause after age 55 years; no pregnancy prior to age 30 years	*Painless lump; breast erythema; nipple discharge; nipple retraction; skin of breast retracts	Biopsy; mammography	Stage 1: 80–95%, 5-year; 62–73%, 10-year. Stage 2: 71%, 5-year; 53%, 10-year. Stage 3: 40%, 5-year; 31%, 10-year. Stage 4: 25%, 5-year

Cancer	Risk Factors	Signs and Symptoms	Diagnostic Tests	Survival
Central Nervous System Metastases: lung	Age >60 years; white race; industrial workers working with rubber, hydrocarbons, or petroleum; male sex	*Headache; personality changes; seizures; vomiting	CT scan; EEG; MRI; PET	25%, 2-year

Cancer	Risk Factors	Signs and Symptoms	Diagnostic Tests	Survival
Cervix Metastases: bone, bowel, kidney, liver, lung, nodes	Age 20–30 years; age 45–65 years; early age coitus; herpes simplex virus II; residence in Cali, Colombia; multiple sexual partners; repeated douching; smoking	*Bloody discharge; pelvic pain; thin vaginal discharge	Colposcopy; conization; endocervical curettage; Pap test	In situ: 100% curable. Stage 1: 90%, 5-year. Stage 2: 65%, 5-year. Stage 3: 30%, 5-year. Stage 4: 12%, 5-year

Cancer	Risk Factors	Signs and Symptoms	Diagnostic Tests	Survival
Colon Metatases: liver, lung, nodes	Age 20–70 years; diet high in charcoal-broiled or fried foods; diet high in fat or cholesterol; diet low in fiber; living in North America, Western Europe, Scotland, Australia, or New Zealand; ulcerative colitis or polyp history	*Bleeding rectally; abdominal pain; change in bowel pattern; weight loss	BE; CEA; chest radiograph; colonoscopy; CT, liver and spleen; digital examination; occult blood in stool; sigmoidoscopy	In situ: 100% curable; Stage 1: 85%, 5-year. Stage 2: 70%, 5-year. Stage 3: 45–60%, 5-year. Stage 4: 3%, 5-year

Cancer	Risk Factors	Signs and Symptoms	Diagnostic Tests	Survival
Endometrium Metastases: bone, bowel, kidney, lung, nodes	Age >60 years; white race; early menarche; estrogen replacement therapy in post menopause period; high socioeconomic status; late menopause; no children; obesity	*Bleeding; bloating; pain	Biopsy; endocervical curettage	50%, 5-year

Cancer	Risk Factors	Signs and Symptoms	Diagnostic Tests	Survival
Esophagus Metastases: adrenals, bone, liver, lung, nodes	Age 50–60 years; residence in East or South Africa, Iraq, Iran, or northern China; male sex; smoking combined with alcohol intake	*Dysphagia; cough; epigastric pain; vocal cord paralysis; weight loss	Barium esophagogram; biopsy; CT, chest; esophagoscopy	10%, 5-year

Cancer	Risk Factors	Signs and Symptoms	Diagnostic Tests	Survival
Gallbladder Metastases: liver, nodes	Age >65 years; female sex; gallstones; Hispanic; residence in Israel, Europe, Japan, Latin America; many pregnancies	*Abdominal pain; nausea; vomiting; weight loss	BE; biopsy; CEA; CT scan; MRI	10%, 5-year

Cancer	Risk Factors	Signs and Symptoms	Diagnostic Tests	Survival
Head and Neck Metastases: lung, nodes, skin	Age >40 years; alcohol abuse; chronic irritation: poorly fitting dentures; Epstein-Barr virus; iron deficiency; male sex; tobacco abuse; sunlight exposure	*Pain; dysphagia; hoarseness; weight loss	Biopsy; chest radiograph; CT scan; endoscopic examination; MRI; visual inspection of oral cavity	Stage 1: 30–40% cured. Stage 4: rarely cured

Cancer	Risk Factors	Signs and Symptoms	Diagnostic Tests	Survival
Hodgkin's Disease Metastases: liver, lung, nodes, spleen	Age, early 20's; Age, late 70's; ataxia; telangiectasia; Epstein-Barr virus; well-educated	*Lymph node enlargement; fatigue; night sweats; itching; weight loss	Biopsy; CBC; chest radiograph; CT, chest; SMA-20	80%, 5-year

Cancer	Risk Factors	Signs and Symptoms	Diagnostic Tests	Survival
Kidney Metastases: bone, brain, liver, lung, nodes	Age 58–64 years; family history of renal cancer; history of von Hippel–Lindau disease; residence in North America or northern Europe; male sex; obesity; tobacco abuse	*Hematuria; abdominal pain; anemia; bloating, abdomen; nausea; weight loss	Biopsy; CT, abdomen; inferior venacavography; IVP; MRI; renal angiography or ultrasonography; urinalysis	Local disease: 60–80%, 5-year. Extension: 50%, 5-year. Lymph nodes: 15–20%, 5-year. Metastasis: 5%, 5-year

Cancer	Risk Factors	Signs and Symptoms	Diagnostic Tests	Survival
Larynx Metastases: lung, nodes, skin	Age >58 years; black race; smoking cigarettes; exposure to tobacco, nickel, alcohol, asbestos, and mustard gas; heavy alcohol consumption; male sex	*Hoarseness; bloody sputum; sore throat; swallowing problems	Biopsy; chest radiograph; endoscopic examination; visual inspection of oral cavity	Stage 1: high cure. Stage 4: 1-year

Cancer	Risk Factors	Signs and Symptoms	Diagnostic Tests	Survival
Leukemia in Children Metastases: brain, lung, meninges	Age 2–6 years; benzene exposure; Down's syndrome; family history of leukemia; human T-cell leukemia virus; ionizing radiation exposure; Philadelphia chromosome	*Fever; joint pain; membrane bleeding; organ enlargement of spleen, lymphatics, or liver; pallor	Bone marrow aspiration; CBC; lumbar puncture	Acute lymphocytic leukemia (ALL): 50%, 5-year. WBC <10,000, survival is 85%, 5-year. WBC >40,000, survival is 40%, 5-year. Acute non-lymphocytic leukemia (ANLL): 20%, 5-year

Cancer	Risk Factors	Signs and Symptoms	Diagnostic Tests	Survival
Leukemia in Adults Metastases: brain, lung, meninges	Exposure to radioactive fallout; Fanconi's syndrome; heredity of leukemia; non-Asian persons	*Fatigue; bruising; fever; joint pain; organ enlargement of spleen, lymphatics, or liver; pallor; repeated infections	Bone marrow aspiration; CBC	Acute lymphocytic leukemia (ALL): 40–80% remission rate (RR), 12–26 month mean survival (MMS). Acute myelogenous leukemia (AML): 50–70% RR, 15–18 MMS. Chronic myelogenous leukemia (CML): 10% RR, 1–6 MMS. Chronic lymphocytic leukemia (CLL). 40–60% RR, 12–28 MMS

Cancer	Risk Factors	Signs and Symptoms	Diagnostic Tests	Survival
Liver Metastases: colon, lung	Cirrhosis; exposure to multiple venereal diseases, illicit drugs, aflatoxins; hepatitis-B virus; residence in Mozambique, China, or Japan	*Pain, RUQ abdomen; ascites; jaundice; liver enlargement	AFP; biopsy; CT, liver; liver function tests	Stage 1: 3 years. Stage 2: 7 months. Stage 3: 3 months

Cancer	Risk Factors	Signs and Symptoms	Diagnostic Tests	Survival
Lung Metastases: bone, brain, kidney, liver, marrow, meninges, nodes, skin	Age >55 years; asbestos exposure; hydrocarbon or chemical exposure; residence in western Europe or North America; passive smoke inhalation; smoking	*Cough; *dyspnea; changes in sputum; hemoptysis; malaise; weight loss	Biopsy; bone marrow aspiration; bone scan; bronchial washing; brushing cytology; CBC; chest radiograph with PA and lat.; CT, lung; liver profile, serum; sputum cytology	Non–small cell = Stage 1: 65%, 2-year; 50%, 5-year. Stage 2: 30%, 5-year. Stage 3: 10%, 5-year. Stage 4: 1%, 5-year; 20%, 1-year

Cancer	Risk Factors	Signs and Symptoms	Diagnostic Tests	Survival
Lymphoma, Non–Hodgkin's Metastases: brain, lung, meninges	Age >50 years; excessive radiation exposure; residence in city; nickel or chromium exposure	*Lymph node enlargement, painless; *night sweats; bone pain; fever; history of lymphadenopathy; pruritus; weight loss	Biopsy; bone marrow aspiration; bone scan; CBC; chest radiograph; CT, abdomen; liver scan; SMA-20	60–80% curable; survival 65%, 3-year

Cancer	Risk Factors	Signs and Symptoms	Diagnostic Tests	Survival
Melanoma Metastases: bone, brain, liver, lung, nodes, skin	Age >40 years; white race; first-degree relative with melanoma; heritage with red or blond hair and blue eyes; history of intermittent intense sun exposure during childhood; precursor to melanocytic lesion; sunburned skin	*Asymmetrically shaped lesion; bleeding lesion; color disparity of lesion; irregular borders of lesion	Biopsy; bone marrow aspiration; chest radiograph; CT scan; hemogram; liver function tests	65–75%, 5-year. Regional lymph node metastasis: 15–50%, 5-year. Distant metastasis: 5–18 months

Cancer	Risk Factors	Signs and Symptoms	Diagnostic Tests	Survival
Multiple Myeloma Metastases: lung, nodes	Age >60 years; fair skin; family history; male sex	*Bone pain; lymph-adenopathy	Bone marrow aspiration; sedimentation rate, blood; serum electrophoresis, M component; urinalysis for protein; radiograph, skeletal; radiograph, skull	Large tumor mass: weeks or months. Rarity: 20 years

Cancer	Risk Factors	Signs and Symptoms	Diagnostic Tests	Survival
Neuroblastoma Metastases: bone, brain	Age <6 years; chromosomal abnormality of 1p, 1q, 17q; von Recklinghausen's disease	*Enlarged abdomen; anorexia; bone pain; diarrhea; Horner's syndrome; irritability; limping	Bone marrow aspiration; bone scan; chest radiograph; CT, chest/abdominal; IVP; NSE tumor marker, serum; nuclear imaging with MIBG; ultrasound of abdomen; urine, HVA; urine VMA	<1 year old: 70% long-term. Stage 1: 60%, 5-year. Stage 2: 30%, 5-year. Stage 3: 15%, 5-year. Stage 4: 3%, 5-year

Cancer	Risk Factors	Signs and Symptoms	Diagnostic Tests	Survival
Oral Cavity Metastases: lung, nodes, skin	Age >45 years; alcohol abuse; American Indian; male sex; poor nutrition; job as farmer, leather worker, printer, or paper manufacturer; ill-fitting dentures; tobacco use	*Soreness in the mouth; bleeding in the mouth; dysphagia; weight loss	Biopsy; CT scan; visual inspection of the oral cavity	10–20%, 5-year

Cancer	Risk Factors	Signs and Symptoms	Diagnostic Tests	Survival
Ovary Metastases: bowel, liver, lung, nodes	Asbestos or talc exposure; early menopause; high-fat diet; infertility; nulliparity; pelvic irradiation	*Vague GI complaint; abdominal bloating; anorexia; dyspepsia; early satiety; flatulence	BE; IVP; OCA-125 antigen, serum; ultrasound of pelvis; upper GI	20%, 5-year; 60%, 2-year

Cancer	Risk Factors	Signs and Symptoms	Diagnostic Tests	Survival
Pancreas Metastases: bowel, liver, lung, nodes	Age >40 years; black race; chronic pancreatitis; smoking cigarettes; diabetes mellitus in females; Jewish; male sex; workers in coke plant or with glass or chemicals	*Jaundice; anorexia; upper abdominal pain; weight loss	Amylase, serum; CBC; CT scan; ERCP; glucose, blood; liver function tests; occult blood in stool; PTC; PTT; ultrasound; upper GI with contrast medium	4%, 5-year. Palliative care for 6–8 months

Cancer	Risk Factors	Signs and Symptoms	Diagnostic Tests	Survival
Prostate Metastases: bone, liver, lung, nodes	Age >50 years; North American; black race; blood relative had prostate cancer; obesity	*Weakness in urinary stream; frequency of urine; lumbar-sacral pain; nocturia	Acid phosphatase, serum; bone scan; CT scan; prostate-specific antigen, blood; rectal examination; ultrasound	5-year: Stage A, 92%; Stage A2, 80%; Stage B, 80%; Stage B2, 30%; Stage C, 25%; Stage D, 10%

Cancer	Risk Factors	Signs and Symptoms	Diagnostic Tests	Survival
Rectum Metastases: colon, liver, lung, nodes	Age >50 years; white race; low-fiber diet; male sex	*Bleeding rectally; rectal pain	BE; colonoscopy; CT of the abdomen/pelvis; digital examination; occult blood in stool; sigmoidoscopy	50%, 5-year

Cancer	Risk Factors	Signs and Symptoms	Diagnostic Tests	Survival
Retinoblastoma Metastases: brain, skin	Age <6 years; family history; tumors are bilateral in 30% of cases; white race	*Eye pain; eye swelling; headache	Biopsy; CT, eye; MRI; visual examination using an ophthalmoscope	20%, 5-year

Cancer	Risk Factors	Signs and Symptoms	Diagnostic Tests	Survival
Skin, Nonmelanoma Types Metastases: lung, nodes	Age 60–80 years; chronic irritation; hydrocarbon exposure; melanin pigmentation; sun exposure	*Rapid growth of lesion; bleeding of lesion; skin thickening or color changes	Biopsy	95% are curable at time of primary diagnosis

Cancer	Risk Factors	Signs and Symptoms	Diagnostic Tests	Survival
Stomach Metastases: bone, liver, lung, nodes	Age >70 years; black race; blood type A; diet high in nitrates; family history of stomach CA; gastric polyps; residence in Japan, Finland, Iceland, Chile, Colombia, or Costa Rica; male sex; pernicious anemia	*Epigastric pain; anorexia; dysphagia; jaundice; vomiting; weight loss	BE; CEA; endoscopic examination; iron, serum; occult blood in stool; upper GI series	10–15%, overall 5-year. 90%, 5-year if lesions confined to mucosa or submucosa. Penetrating lesions have 50% 5-year survival

Cancer	Risk Factors	Signs and Symptoms	Diagnostic Tests	Survival
Testes Metastases: bone, liver, lung, nodes	Age 20–40 years; atrophic testes; cryptorchid testes; high scrotal temperature; history of leukemia; polythelia syndrome	*Scrotal mass, painless; anorexia; back pain; epididymitis; nausea; scrotal pain	AFP; biopsy; B-subunit HCG; chest radiograph; CT scan; retroperitoneum	Stage 1: 90% cured; Stage 2: 85% cured; Stage 3: 75% cured; Stage 4: 20% cured

Cancer	Risk Factors	Signs and Symptoms	Diagnostic Tests	Survival
Thyroid Metastases: bone, lung, nodes	Age 30–60 years; female sex; residence in North America, Iceland, Israel, Switzerland; radiation exposure to neck	*Lump in neck; difficulty in swallowing; hoarseness	Biopsy; history and physical examination; thyroid scan	80%, 10-year

Cancer	Risk Factors	Signs and Symptoms	Diagnostic Tests	Survival
Uterus Metastases: lung, pelvis	Age 51–60 years; diabetes mellitus; exogenous estrogen use during menopause; family history of ovarian, breast, colon, uterus CA; hypertension; nulliparity; obesity	*Vaginal bleeding; intermenstrual spotting; postcoital bleeding	Biopsy; Pap test	Stage 1: 75%, 5-year; Stage 2: 50%, 5-year; Stage 3: 25%, 5-year; Stage 4: 10%, 5-year

Cancer	Risk Factors	Signs and Symptoms	Diagnostic Tests	Survival
Vagina Metastases: cervix, colon, endometrium, lung, rectum	Age 60–70 years; DES exposure in utero; history of cervical or vulvar cancer	*Vaginal discharge and bleeding; urinary symptoms	Biopsy; colposcopy; history and physical examination; Pap test	In situ: 100% curable; Stage 1: 64%, 5-year; Stages 2, 3, and 4: 50%, 5-year

Cancer	Risk Factors	Signs and Symptoms	Diagnostic Tests	Survival
Vulva Metastases: cervix, nodes, rectum	White race; chronic vulvitis; diabetes mellitus; history of cervical cancer; hypertension; obesity	*Vulvar lump; bloody discharge; groin mass; pruritus	Biopsy using toluidine blue 10% solution	In situ: 100% curable; 70% overall, 5-year

Cancer	Risk Factors	Signs and Symptoms	Diagnostic Tests	Survival
Wilms' Tumor Metastases: lung, liver	Age <7 years; aniridia; Beckwith-Wiedemann syndrome; chromosome deletion of 11p; cryptorchidism	*Abdominal mass; fever, low; hematuria; hypertension; pain in abdomen	CT, abdomen; IVP; ultrasound	88%, 2-year; 8–10%, long-term with no complications in later life

PART II

DIAGNOSTIC TESTS

Acid Phosphatase, Serum. Norms are 1 to 5 King-Armstrong μ/dL, 0.5 to 2 Bodansky or Gutman μ/dL, 0.1 to 0.73 Bessey Lowry μ/nk, 0.1 to 0.63 Sigma units, or 0 to 1.1 Shinowara μ/mL. An enzyme whose primary activity is in the prostate gland, it is also found in bone, liver, spleen, kidney, red blood cells, and platelets. Levels are significantly elevated in cancer of the prostate. When this tumor is treated successfully by surgery, the level will fall within 4 days or within 4 weeks if treated with estrogen therapy.

AFP. Alpha-fetoprotein is a glycoprotein produced in the yolk sac, liver, and gastrointestinal (GI) tract of the fetus and reaches a peak serum concentration of 3 ng/mL at 12 weeks' gestation. This value in adulthood ranges from 1 to 25 ng/mL. The value is elevated in persons who are pregnant; in persons with hepatomas or germ cell tumors; and in 25% of persons with GI, pancreatic, or lung cancer.

Amylase, Serum. Norm is 60 to 200 Somogyi u/100 mL. An enzyme produced in the fallopian tubes, liver, pancreas, and salivary glands that changes starch into sugar.

Barium Esophagogram. Use of oral barium contrast to permit visualization of the lumen of the esophagus. The client will be NPO after midnight before the test and remain NPO until the test is completed. First the client will have a preliminary plain film x-ray of the esophagus done. Then the client swallows the chalky barium contrast while standing in front of the fluoroscope. More radiographs are taken, with possible follow-up x-ray films in 24 hours. The procedure takes about 45 minutes. A postprep is to be given to evacuate barium from the bowel.

BE. With barium enema, the colon is examined while fluoroscopy and x-rays are used to assess the position, filling, and movement of the parts of the large intestine. The client, after being bowel prepped the day before and NPO after midnight, lies on his or her back for a preliminary abdominal radiograph. Then, with the client lying on his or her side, the barium is placed into the colon by an enema. The barium is retained, and several spot radiographs are taken. At the completion, the client is asked to go to the bathroom and expel the barium. A postprep is needed to evacuate the barium. The procedure takes about 90 minutes.

Biopsy. Obtaining a sample of tissue or fluid for pathologic examination. The types include bone marrow, breast, cervical, excisional, incisional, needle, prostate, punch, and skin biopsies.

Biopsy Using Toluidine Blue 10% Solution. This solution is a nuclear stain that is painted on the entire vulva and then is washed off after 5 minutes with a 3% acetic acid solution. The areas that remain blue are punch-biopsed using an instrument that works like a small borer drill, taking out a circular 5-mm plug of skin from the anesthetized area.

Bone Marrow Aspiration. Aspiration of a sample of cells active in blood cell production from the sternum, iliac crest, vertebral body, or, in infants, the tibia. The skin is prepared with antiseptic, the area is anesthetized with Xylocaine, and a short stout needle is inserted into the center of the bone. The stylet is withdrawn, a sterile dry 5- to 10-mL needle is attached, and 0.2–0.5 mL of marrow is aspirated. Moderate pain and heavy pressure are felt at the time of aspiration. The specimen is immediately sent to the laboratory, and the site is dressed with a sterile pressure dressing with or without thromboplastin. Then, the client remains flat in bed for 30 minutes.

Bone Scan. Used to evaluate bone pain. Client is asked to urinate prior to test, as a full bladder will mask the pelvic bones. Then he or she is injected with radioactive technetium-99m phosphate intravenously. This substance mimics calcium physiologically and concentrates more heavily in bone undergoing abnormal changes, leading to "hot spots" on the scan. The client is then asked to drink 1 to 6 glasses of water. After a 2-hour postinjection waiting period, the scanning is done by moving the table on which the client lies under and over a sensitive radiation detector. The scan takes 30 to 60 minutes to complete.

Bronchial Washings. NPO 2 hours prior to test. After the insertion of a fiberoptic bronchoscope, normal saline is instilled, and the residue is gathered for cytologic examination.

Brushings Cytology. NPO 2 hours prior to the test. After the insertion of a fiberoptic bronchoscope, a small brush is inserted and rotated to gather specimens for cytologic examination.

B-Subunit HCG. A hormone that is produced in the presence of active chorionic villi, which can occur during the conditions of pregnancy, hydatidiform mole, choriocarcinoma of the uterus, or testicular seminoma.

CBC. Complete blood count consists of multiple tests run on a single 7-mL blood sample. These tests give valuable information regarding diagnosis, prognosis, and response to treatment. The CBC includes white blood cell count (WBC), differential white blood cell count (Diff), red blood cell count (RBC), hematocrit (Hct), hemoglobin (Hgb), platelet count (Plt), a stained red blood cell examination of a blood smear, and three red blood cell indices that include mean corpuscular volume (MCV), mean corpuscular hemoglobin (MCH), and mean corpuscular hemoglobin concentration (MCHC).

CEA. Carcinoembryonic antigen is a cell surface glycoprotein that increases in production in response to many types of cancer and benign diseases such as inflammatory bowel, liver, renal, pulmonary, or collagen diseases, and in heavy smokers. The normal value for CEA is 0 to 5 ng/mL.

Chest Radiograph. Radiographic picture of the chest while the client is in an upright position so fluid levels can be better detected. The client is asked to take a deep breath and hold it for several seconds while the picture is being taken. Two views of the chest, front view (PA) and side view (lat.), are usually taken. The procedure takes only a few minutes.

Colonoscopy. Examination of 60 cm of the large intestine with a long fiberoptic instrument. A bowel prep consisting of laxatives and enemas is administered during the 24 hours prior to the test, and the client remains on a clear liquid diet until he or she is NPO after midnight. Light sedation is given prior to the examination, the client placed on his or her left side, the rectum dilated, and the scope inserted using air pumped in to distend the intestinal walls for better visualization. The examination takes from 30 minutes to 2 hours.

Colposcopy. Visualization of the vagina and cervix with 5 to 50 times magnification using a telescope-type instrument called a colposcope. A speculum is inserted into the vagina. A cotton applicator is used to dry the cervix, and 3% acetic acid solution is applied to dissolve mucus and to sharpen visibility to distinguish normal from abnormal squamous epithelium. Biopsies or photographs are taken, the speculum is removed, and a pad or tampon is used to absorb the small amount of postprocedural vaginal bleeding.

Conization. Surgical removal of part of the cervix using a scalpel or carbon dioxide laser as the result of a positive biopsy for severe dysplasia or cancer in situ.

CT Scan. Computed tomography is a radiographic study that provides cross-sectional views of soft tissue by passing multiple x-ray beams through the body at different angles and then restructuring the information in the shape of a picture by using a computer. CT may be done with or without a contrast agent. The client is placed in a large circular chamber and is asked to lie perfectly still while the machine moves to take pictures for a total of 30 minutes to 3 hours if the total body is scanned.

Cystoscopy. Viewing of the interior of the bladder and urethra using a tubular lighted telescope. The client's genitalia are scrubbed with antiseptic. Then the client is placed in the lithotomy position, a local anesthetic jelly is placed in the urethra, and the cystoscope inserted for the 15-minute examination.

Digital Examination. Examination of a body part or organ by using a lubricated gloved finger for purposes of using touch to detect abnormalities.

EEG. Electroencephalography is the electrical measurement of brain impulses. The client has 16 to 25 electrodes placed on his or her head using conduction paste or a cap and is instructed to close his or her eyes and relax. A machine in another room will then run for 30 to 45 minutes printing out the brain impulses.

Endocervical Curettage. Scraping of the lining of the cervix. The female client is placed in the lithotomy position, an anesthetic is given, a speculum is inserted, and the cervix is scraped.

Endoscopic Examination. Examination of a body part or system using an optic type instrument with magnification powers and often a lighted source. Specific preparations are often necessary prior to the examination.

ERCP. Endoscopic retrograde cholangiopancreatography is the radiographic examination of the pancreatic ducts and hepatobiliary tree after injection of contrast medium into the duodenal papilla. The person is NPO after midnight. An I.V. line is started, and local anesthetic and intravenous sedative are given. The endoscope is passed down the throat, contrast medium is injected, and x-ray films are taken. Tissue specimens are withdrawn if desired, and the endoscope is then removed. The procedure takes 1 hour. No food or liquids are permitted for 2 hours or until the gag reflex returns.

Esophagoscopy. A flexible fiberoptic endoscope is used to visualize the internal structures of the esophagus. The person is NPO after midnight. An I.V. line is started, and a sedative, analgesic, and local anesthetic are given. The scope is passed to the esophagus, where visualization occurs. Then pictures or biopsies can be taken. The procedure takes 1 hour.

Glucose, Blood. Norms are 60 to 110 mg/dL. Collect 5 mL of blood in a gray-top tube. Glucose is a sugar that is formed from dietary carbohydrate and is also released as a by-product of cells. It is stored as glycogen in the liver and skeletal muscles, where it is ready for the process of gluconeogenesis. This laboratory value is often elevated in persons with cancer.

Hemogram. Common hematologic tests evaluated by automated methods from one 7-mL sample of blood. These tests include the WBC, RBC, Hgb, Hct, MCV, MCHC, MCH, red blood cell distribution width (RDW), and platelet count. Adding a WBC differential count and RBC and platelet morphology to a hemogram produces the test called a complete blood count (CBC).

History and Physical Examination. Data gathering about an individual through asking questions that pertain to his or her health (history) and employing hands-on examination techniques (physical examination) in efforts to aid in diagnosis and treatment.

Inferior Venacavography. Radiographs taken to determine the patency of the venous system and to detect masses in the renal veins. The client is given a bowel prep and is NPO after midnight. Sedative is administered. Contrast material is injected into the inferior vena cava via the femoral vein, and then radiographs are taken. The procedure takes 45 minutes.

Iron, Serum. The norm is 50 to 150 μg (mcg) or 10 to 27 μmol/L (SI units). A venous blood sample of 5 to 10 mL is drawn into a red-top tube. Iron is necessary to synthesize hemoglobin that is essential to transport oxygen to blood cells and tissues. The following medications may cause false values for serum iron: chloramphenicol, ACTH, iron supplements, or oral contraceptives.

IVP. Intravenous urography is a radiographic examination of the kidneys. The client is given a bowel prep and is NPO after midnight. A KUB (kidney, bladder, bowel) plain abdominal x-ray film is taken. Then radiopaque iodine dye is injected intravenously, and further radiographs are taken. The procedure takes 45 minutes. Prior to the procedure, assess for a history of hypersensitivity to iodine, shellfish, or contrast medium with iodine. The client may experience a burning sensation when the dye is injected, as well as a metallic taste.

Liver Function Tests. Tests of blood, urine, and stool to determine the amount and distribution of bile pigments; blood tests to demonstrate liver function; and blood tests to determine the liver's excretory functions or presence of hepatic damage.

Liver Profile, Serum. Serum test to detect amount of bilirubin in the blood. The norm is 0 to 0.02 mg/dL. Bilirubin is a by-product of hemoglobin that is excreted into the GI tract and is broken down by bacteria into urobilinogen when it is excreted by the liver and urinary system. The client should fast 4 hours prior to the test.

Liver Scan. Radiographic study of the liver to determine the level of dysfunction. No prep is given. A technetium compound is administered intravenously, the person waits 15 minutes, then the liver is scanned by x-rays as the client lies as still as possible. The procedure takes 30 minutes to 1 hour. Do not schedule the liver scan if another radioactive scan has been done within 24 hours, as trace amounts of radioactivity may exist.

Lower GI Series. Otherwise known as a barium enema (BE), radiographic examination of the large intestine.

Lumbar Puncture. Obtaining cerebrospinal fluid sample for the purpose of examining the fluid within the spinal cord. The client lies on his or her side, with the knees drawn up as far as possible and head bent down toward the chest. Between the third and fourth lumbar vertebrae the area is cleansed with antiseptic, a local anesthetic is administered, and a needle is inserted that causes transient pain. Then 5 to 10 mL of fluid is withdrawn into two or three tubes, and a dry sterile pressure dressing is applied over the puncture site. The total procedure takes 20 minutes. A headache is a common side effect that may last for several hours. The client is to lie flat for 8 hours after the test.

Mammography. Radiographic examination of the breast that detects cysts and tumors. No prep is necessary. The client removes clothes and jewelry from the neck to the waist. Then the breast is compressed between plates with only minor discomfort, the client holds his or her breath, and the radiograph is taken. The procedure takes 15 to 30 minutes.

Monoclonal Antibodies. Antibodies produced by a single clone of B-lymphocytes that are directed against an antigen on a tumor cell.

MRI. Magnetic resonance imaging uses magnetic fields and radiowaves to create images of soft tissue, muscle, fat, and internal organs. Clients must remove all metallic objects and inform the technologist if they have any prosthetics (clips, plates, joints, pacemaker, implanted venous access devices) or are pregnant. The client must lie still while in a semi-enclosed scanner for 30 to 60 minutes.

NSE Tumor Marker, Serum. Neuron-specific enolase is the brain neuronal form of the glycolytic enzyme enolase that is present in peripheral and neuroendocrine cells. The norm is less than 20 ng/mL. Increased serum levels are found in persons with neuroblastoma or small cell carcinoma of the lung.

Nuclear Imaging with MIBG. Nuclear imaging test using meta-iodobenzyl guanosine to detect neuroblastoma in children.

OCA-125 Antigen, Serum. Antigen found in the blood of persons with ovarian cancer. The norm is 0 to 35 U/mL. Useful for monitoring the course of the disease during adjuvant therapies.

Occult Blood, Stool. Testing for nonvisible blood in the stool by using a commercial occult test kit. The client should avoid ingesting meats, poultry, fish, and beets for 3 days prior to testing.

Pap Test. Papanicolaou smear cytology test of the cervix. The client should not douche, administer vaginal medication, or have sexual intercourse for 24 hours prior to the test. The test should be done between menstrual periods. The client lies in a lithotomy position, and a speculum is inserted into the vagina. Then a curved wooden Pap spatula stick scrapes the cervix in three areas, and the specimen is transferred onto a slide and fixated. The procedure takes 10 minutes.

PET. Positive emission tomography creates images of slices of the brain similar to a CT image.

Prostate-Specific Antigen. A peptide found specifically in the prostate that is useful for monitoring therapy and disease progressions of prostate cancer. The norm is less than 4 ng/mL.

PTC. Percutaneous transhepatic cholangiography is a radiographic examination that uses contrast medium injected into the liver for the purpose of assessing an obstructed biliary system. The person is NPO after midnight prior to the test. The percutaneous catheter can be left in place to provide for biliary decompression. The procedure takes 1 hour.

PTT. Partial thromboplastin time is a blood test that detects deficiencies in intrinsic clotting factors (except factors VII and XIII) and in platelet variations. It is also useful for monitoring heparin therapy. Collect a 7-mL venous blood sample in a blue-top tube. The norm is 30 to 45 seconds.

Radiograph, Bone. Noninvasive radiographic film of the bone useful for assessing metastasis and pathologic fractures.

Radiograph, Skeletal. Noninvasive radiographic film of the entire body skeleton done to evaluate metastasis and generalized pain.

Radiograph, Skull. Noninvasive radiographic film of the three groups of head bones (vault, jaw, and facial bones) in order to assess metastasis of the skull and increased intracranial pressure.

Rectal Examination. Digital examination and endoscopic examination of the rectum using a 7-cm fiberoptic proctoscope. Specimens may be obtained by biopsy, brushings, or a swab.

Renal Angiography. Radiographic examination of the kidney vasculature and parenchyma after a femoral arterial injection of iodine contrast medium. The client is NPO after midnight. Any metal objects should be removed from the client's body. Then an analgesic and sedative are given, and radiographs are taken. The procedure takes 1 hour. Post-testing care includes lying flat for 8 hours.

Renal Ultrasonography. High-frequency sound waves are transmitted through the kidneys, resulting in echos that are amplified and converted into electrical impulses and displayed on an oscilloscope screen. The client lies in the prone position. Ultrasound jelly is applied, and the transducer is moved over the kidney area as the client takes a deep breath in order to assess the kidneys during respiration. The procedure takes 30 minutes.

Sedimentation Rate, Blood. The rate at which RBCs settle in unclotted blood in millimeters per hour. In males, the rate is 0 to 10 mm/hr; in females, 0 to 20 mm/hr. Increases in infections and malignancies. Obtain a 7-mL venous blood sample in a lavender-top tube.

Serum Electrophoresis, M Component. Blood serum is placed on specially treated paper that is exposed to electrical current so specific patterns can develop. Gamma-globulins from multiple myeloma cause patterns that spike and resemble the letter "M."

Sigmoidoscopy. Examination of the anus, rectum, and sigmoid colon using a 25- to 30-cm fiberoptic sigmoidoscope or a 60-cm flexible scope to visualize the descending colon. The client is prepped with laxatives and enemas and is NPO after midnight. The scope is inserted, and air is injected to better visualize the structures by spreading the intestinal walls apart. Biopsies may be taken. The procedure takes 30 minutes.

SMA-20. The sequential multiple analyzer is an automated machine that electronically determines 20 different serologic tests from one 10-mL specimen of blood in 1 hour. The tests include profiles on electrolytes, lipids, and renal, hepatic, and cardiac systems.

Sputum Cytology. A sterile sample of sputum is sent to the laboratory to investigate abnormalities in the color, size, and shape of cell substances.

Thyroid Scan. Radioactive iodine is given intravenously or in liquid or capsule form orally. Then the client waits for a period of approximately 30 minutes, at which time radiographs are taken of the thyroid region. Three days prior to the test, the client should discontinue ingestion of iodine salt, thyroid hormones, corticosteroids, aspirin, phenothiazines, seafood, and multivitamins. The client should be NPO after midnight prior to the test.

Ultrasound. Noninvasive diagnostic procedure used to visualize body tissue structures. A transducer is held over the client's skin surface that produces an ultrasound beam to the tissues, which is then recorded on an oscilloscope.

Upper GI Series. Fluoroscopic and x-ray examination of the esophagus, stomach, and small intestine using oral barium as a contrast medium. The client is NPO after midnight. The procedure takes 1 to 4 hours. Postprep laxative is needed to help expel the barium.

Urinalysis. Preferred first-morning 10-mL urine sample that is assessed in the laboratory for color, odor, appearance, pH, sugars, epithelial cells, casts, crystals, and yeast cells.

Urine HVA. Homovanillic acid is a metabolite of dopamine, a major catecholamine that is found in the urine of persons that have neuroblastoma or ganglioneuroma. The norm is less than 8 mg/24 hr. Collect a 24-hour urine in a plastic bottle with preservative.

Urine VMA. Vanillylmandelic acid is a major by-product of the catecholamines epinephrine and norepinephrine. High urine levels indicate an adrenal tumor. The norms are 1.5 to 7.5 mg/24 hr or 7.6 to 37.9 μmol/24 hr (SI units). Collect a 24-hour urine in a plastic bottle with preservative.

Visual Inspection of Oral Cavity. Visual assessment of the oral mucosa, palates, tongue, teeth, and gums for abnormalities.

X-ray. *See* radiograph.

PART III

CHEMOTHERAPEUTIC AGENTS

L-Asparaginase (L-ASP, Elspar)

Please tell the nurse or doctor if you have any of the following:

1. Chills
2. Fever
3. Hives
4. Nausea or vomiting
5. Nosebleed

L-ASPARAGINASE (L-ASP, ELSPAR)

Drug Action	Side Effects	Special Considerations	Cancers Effective Against
Enzyme that breaks down the amino acid asparagine	Anaphylaxis	Risk increases with drug usage	Acute lymphocytic leukemia (ALL)
	Chills	Common	
	CNS depression	Rare	
	Fever	Common	
	Hemorrhage	Rare	
	Hepatotoxicity	Common within 2 weeks	
	Hyperglycemia	Occasional	
	Nausea/vomiting	Moderate/severe	
	Pancreatitis	Occasional	
	Renal toxicity	Common	
	Weight loss	Rare	

Bleomycin Sulfate (Bleo, BLENOXANE)

Please tell the nurse or doctor if you have any of the following:

1. Poor appetite
2. Breathing difficulty
3. Fatigue
4. Fever
5. Hair loss
6. Mouth sores
7. Possible pregnancy
8. Skin that is itchy, red, or peeling

BLEOMYCIN SULFATE (Bleo, BLENOXANE)

Drug Action	Side Effects	Special Considerations	Cancers Effective Against
Antibiotic that is cell cycle–nonspecific and binds directly to DNA, causing decreased synthesis of DNA, RNA, and proteins, which leads to cellular destruction	Alopecia	Starts 3–4 weeks	Cervical; choriocarcinoma; germ cell; head and neck; Hodgkin's disease; lung; lymphoma; melanoma; penis; sarcoma; testicular; vulva
	Anaphylaxis	Mostly lymphoma	
	Anorexia	Can be severe	
	Fatigue	Can be severe	
	Fever	103–105°F common 3–6 hr after therapy	
	Hyperpigmentation	Nails, joints, pressure points get red/yellow	
Nadir = 7–10 days	Mutagenic	?Teratogenic	
	Photosensitivity	Use sunblock	
	Pulmonary	Pneumonitis with fine rales, fibrosis if cum. dose > 400 U	
	Radiation recall	Use sunblockers	
	Renal toxicity	Decrease dose if creatinine >1.5 mg/dL	
	Skin changes	Peeling, pruritus, ulcerations	
	Stomatitis	Moderate	
	Ulcerations	Hands	

Busulfan (BUS, MYLERAN)

Please tell the nurse or doctor if you have any of the following:

1. Breast enlargement
2. Breathing difficulty
3. Fatigue
4. Hair thinning
5. Hazy vision
6. Menstrual period problems
7. Nausea or vomiting
8. Skin color changes

BUSULFAN   (BUS, Myleran)

Drug Action	Side Effects	Special Considerations	Cancers Effective Against
Alkylating agent that causes alkylation of DNA and sulfhydryl groups, which strips sulfur-containing amino acids, polypeptides, and proteins	Alopecia. . . . . Rare Amenorrhea. . . . . Occasional Cataract . . . . Rare Gynecomastia . . . . Occasional Hyperpigmentation . . . . . Occasional Myelosuppression . . . . . . Moderate, cumulative Nausea/vomiting. . . . . . . Occasional Pulmonary . . . . Fibrosis with prolonged use		Chronic granulocytic leukemia (CGL); chronic myelogenous leukemia (CML)
Nadir = 14–21 days	Sterility. . . . . Dose dependent		

Carboplatin (PARAPLATIN)

Please tell the nurse or doctor if you have any of the following:

1. Breathing difficulty
2. Chest pain
3. Diarrhea
4. Ringing ears
5. Fatigue
6. Hair thinning
7. Hives
8. Nausea or vomiting
9. Numbness or tingling in hands or feet
10. Skin itchy
11. Skin rash
12. Taste malfunction: foods taste metallic

Carboplatin

CARBOPLATIN (Paraplatin)

Drug Action	Side Effects	Special Considerations	Cancers Effective Against
Alkylating agent that reacts with nucleophilic sites on DNA causing intra- or interstrand cross-links rather than DNA-protein cross-links	Alopecia	Rare	Ovarian
	Anaphylaxis	Rare	
	Anemia	Cumulative	
	Constipation	Rare	
	Diarrhea	Occasional	
	Hypersensitivity	2% of all persons	
	Liver dysfunction	5 to 24%, reversible	
	Metallic taste	Occasional	
Nadir = 21 days	Myelosuppression	Dose related	
	Nausea/vomiting	Mild, vomiting may occur 6–12 hours after teatment	
	Neurotoxicity	Rare, 4% of all persons	
	Renal toxicity	Rare	
	Tinnitus	Rare	

Carmustine. (BCNU, BiCNU)

Please tell the nurse or doctor if you have any of the following:

1. Poor appetite
2. Bleeding or bruising
3. Breathing difficulty
4. Confusion at times
5. Diarrhea
6. Flushed face
7. Fatigue
8. Hair loss
9. Mouth sores
10. Nausea or vomiting

Carmustine

Carmustine   (BCNU, BiCNU)
Must be refrigerated and protected from light.

Drug Action	Side Effects	Special Considerations	Cancers Effective Against
Nitrosourea, cell cycle–nonspecific (CCNS) agent that breaks DNA strands and inhibits DNA repair Nadir = 3–6 weeks	Alopecia	Rare	Acute myelogenous leukemia (AML); acute granulocytic leukemia (AGL); central nervous system involvement; gastric; glioma; hepatocellular; Hodgkin's disease; lymphoma; melanoma; multiple myeloma; mycosis fungoides
	Anorexia	Mild	
	Diarrhea	Mild	
	Face flushed	Caused by rapid infusion	
	Hepatotoxic	20% of all cases	
	Hyperpigmentation	Only with direct drug contact	
	Irritant	2–6 mL sodium bicarbonate subcutaneously	
	Leukopenia	5–6 weeks	
	Nausea/vomiting	Severe initially, decreases with subsequent doses	
	Neurotoxicity	Rare	
	Pulmonary	Prolonged use causes pulmonary fibrosis	
	Thrombocytopenia	4–5 weeks	
	Renal toxicity	Occasional	
	Stomatitis	Rare	
	Thrombophlebitis, chemical	Common in several days	

Chlorambucil (CHL, CLB, LEUKERAN)

Please tell the nurse or doctor if you have any of the following:

1. Breathing difficulty
2. Fatigue
3. Nausea and vomiting
4. Skin that is itchy, red, or peeling

Chlorambucil

CHLORAMBUCIL   (CHL, CLB, LEUKERAN)

Drug Action	Side Effects	Special Considerations	Cancers Effective Against
Alkylating agent that interferes with DNA cross-linking replication and transcription	Dermatitis	Occasional	Breast; choriocarcinoma; chronic lymphocytic leukemia (CLL); Hodgkin's disease; lymphoma; multiple myeloma; ovarian; prostate; sarcoma
	Hepatotoxicity	Rare	
	Myelosuppression	Moderate	
	Nausea/vomiting	High doses only	
	Pulmonary	Fibrosis with prolonged use	
Nadir = 7–21 days	Sterility	Occasional	

Chlorotrianisene (TACE)

Please tell the nurse or doctor if you have any of the following:

1. Acne
2. Breast enlargement
3. Chest pain
4. Depressed mood
5. Dizziness
6. Impotence
7. Leg cramps
8. Nausea or vomiting
9. Skin turns yellow
10. Swelling in the calves or redness of the calves of the legs
11. Thirst and greater liquid consumption than usual

Chlorotrianisene

CHLOROTRIANISENE (TACE)
Contraindicated in thromboembolic disorders.

Drug Action	Side Effects	Special Considerations	Cancers Effective Against
Estrogen that increases DNA, RNA, and protein synthesis. Reduces FSH and LH release from the pituitary	Acne	Occasional	Prostate
	Depression	Rare	
	Dizziness	Rare	
	Gynecomastia	Dose dependent	
	Hypercalcemia	Rare	
	Hyperglycemia	Occasional	
	Impotence	Dose dependent	
	Jaundice	Rare	
	Leg cramps	Rare	
	Myocardial infarction	Rare	
	Nausea/vomiting	Occasional	
	Pulmonary emboli	Rare	
	Thromboembolism	Rare	

Cisplatin (CDDP, Diamminedichloroplatinum, DDP, Platinol)

Please tell the nurse or doctor if you have any of the following:

1. Bleeding or bruising
2. Breathing difficulty
3. Diarrhea
4. Ringing ears
5. Swollen face
6. Hearing difficulty
7. Hives
8. Nausea or vomiting
9. Numbness or tingling in hands or feet
10. Taste malfunction: foods taste metallic
11. Urination problems

Cisplatin

CISPLATIN   (CDDP, Diamminedichloroplatinum, DDP, PLATINOL)
Administration of DDP in 3% saline and extensive hydration with NS plus KCl protects against renal damage.

Drug Action	Side Effects	Special Considerations	Cancers Effective Against
Alkylating cell cycle–nonspecific agent that damages DNA and interferes with RNA transcription	Anaphylaxis	1–20% of all cases	Bladder; cervical; endometrial; esophagus; germ cell; head and neck; kidney; lung; lymphoma; ovarian; prostate; sarcoma; testicular
	Bone marrow depression	High doses cause leukopenia and thrombocytopenia	
	Diarrhea	Mild, rare	
	Hyperuricemia	Occasional, responds to the drug allopurinol	
Nadir = 7–14 days	Magnesium wasting	Common with neuromuscular irritability	
	Nausea/vomiting	Controlled with Reglan (metoclopromide hydrochloride)	
	Neurotoxicity	Rare peripheral neuropathies	
	Ototoxicity	Cumulative, may be permanent	
	Renal toxicity	Cumulative, dose limiting	
	Taste changes	Metallic taste to food is common	

Colony-Stimulating Factor (G-CSF, GM-CSF, M-CSF)

Please tell the nurse or doctor if you have any of the following:

1. Bleeding from anywhere on the body
2. Breathing difficulty
3. Chills
4. Diarrhea
5. Flushed face
6. Fatigue
7. Fever
8. Flu-like symptoms
9. Headache
10. Nausea or vomiting
11. Pain in bones

Colony-Stimulating Factor

COLONY-STIMULATING FACTOR (G-CSF, GM-CSF, M-CSF)
Given intravenously or subcutaneously.

Drug Action	Side Effects	Special Considerations	Cancers Effective Against
Cytokines that regulate the growth of stem cells found in the bone marrow Not directly tumoricidal but decrease the duration of neutropenia and enhance the recovery time from myelosuppression	Bone aches . . . . Mild/moderate Diarrhea. . . . . Mild Face flushed . . . . Moderate Flu-like syndrome . . . . . . Occasional Headache . . . . Mild Myelosuppression . . . . . . Moderate Nausea/vomiting. . . . . . . Mild Pulmonary . . . . Rare breathing difficulty	Chronic lymphocytic leukemia; (CLL); hairy cell leukemia; leukemia

Cyclophosphamide (CYTOXAN, CTX, CYT, ENDOXANA, NEOSAR, PROCYTOX)

Please tell the nurse or doctor if you have any of the following:

1. Poor appetite
2. Breathing difficulty
3. Fever
4. Hair loss
5. Menstrual period missed
6. Nausea or vomiting
7. Possible pregnancy
8. Urination that is painful

Cyclophosphamide

CYCLOPHOSPHAMIDE (Cytoxan, CTX, CYT, Endoxana, Neosar, Procytox)

Drug Action	Side Effects	Special Considerations	Cancers Effective Against
Alkylating cell cycle– nonspecific agent that damages DNA and interferes with RNA transcription Nadir = 7–14 days	Alopecia	Regrowth during therapy is 50%	Acute granuloytic leukemia (AGL); acute lymphocytic leukemia (ALL); bladder; breast; bronchogenic; chronic granulocytic leukemia (CGL); choriocarcinoma; chronic lymphocytic leukemia (CLL); colon; germ cell; head and neck; Hodgkin's disease; leukemia; lung; lymphoma; multiple myeloma; mycosis fungoides; neuroblastoma; ovarian; prostate; rectal; retinoblastoma; sarcoma; stomach; Wilms' tumor
	Anorexia	Common	
	Bone marrow depression	Leukopenia in 7–10 days	
	CHF	Rare	
	Dizziness	Caused by rapid high infusion	
	Hemorrhagic cystitis	Hematuria with low/high doses	
	Hepatotoxicity	Rare	
	Nausea/vomiting	4–12 hours after therapy, dose related	
	Pneumonitis	Prolonged, continuous usage	
	Pulmonary	Fibrosis is rare	
	Reproduction	Amenorrhea, azospermia, teratogenic	
	Skin reaction	Nail hyperpigmentation	
	Urinary bladder	Occasional fibrosis	

Cytarabine (Ara-C, Arabinosylcytosine, CYTOSAR)

Please tell the nurse or doctor if you have any of the following:

1. Poor appetite
2. Bleeding or bruising
3. Chills
4. Diarrhea
5. Fever
6. Mouth sores
7. Nausea or vomiting
8. Skin rash
9. Throat that is sore or painful

Cytarabine

CYTARABINE   (Ara-C, Arabinosylcytosine, CYTOSAR)

Drug Action	Side Effects	Special Considerations	Cancers Effective Against
Antimetabolite, cell cycle–specific agent that interrupts DNA synthesis by mimicking the building blocks of DNA Nadir = 7–14 days	Anorexia . . . . Bone marrow depression . . . . Diarrhea. . . . . Esophagitis. . . . . Fever/chills . . . . Hepatotoxicity. . . . . Hyperuricemia. . . . . Nausea/vomiting. . . . . . . Neurotoxicity. . . . . Skin rash . . . . Stomatitis.	Common Begins 4–7 days, recovery 3 weeks Rare Mild Also mild headache 8 hr later Rare Controlled with the drug allopurinol Mild, dose dependent Common with intrathecal use Sensitivity to sun, use sunscreens Mild, common	Acute granulocytic leukemia (AGL); acute lymphocytic leukemia (ALL); acute myelogenous leukemia (AML); blast crisis; chronic granulocytic leukemia (CGL); chronic myelogenous leukemia (CML); central nervous system metastasis; erythroleukemia; Hodgkin's disease; leukemia; lymphoma

Dacarbazine (DTIC, DTIC-DOME, Imidazole Carboxamide)

Please tell the nurse or doctor if you have any of the following:

1. Burning or redness at IV needle site
2. Chills
3. Flushed face
4. Fever
5. Flu-like symptoms
6. Hair thinning
7. Nausea or vomiting
8. Pain or swelling at the IV needle site
9. Possible pregnancy
10. Taste malfunction: foods taste metallic

Dacarbazine

DACARBAZINE   (DTIC, DTIC-DOME, Imidazole Carboxamide)

Protect from light. Change in color from yellow to pink denotes drug decomposition. Precipitates with Solu-Cortef. Potentiates allopurinol.

Drug Action	Side Effects	Special Considerations	Cancers Effective Against
Alkylating cell cycle–nonspecific agent that attaches to DNA, causing misreading of DNA code, which results in cellular death	Alopecia	Moderate	Hodgkin's disease; melanoma; sarcoma
	Anaphylaxis	Rare	
	Anorexia	Mild, metallic taste common	
	Azotemia	Allopurinol potentiated	
	Bone marrow depression	Potentially severe, usually mild	
	Face flushed	Moderate	
	Facial paresthesia	Rare	
Nadir = 10–14 days	Fever/chills	Common	
	Flu syndrome	Common, lasts 7–10 days	
	Hepatotoxicity	Rare	
	Nausea/vomiting	Moderate/severe for 1–2 days	
	Photosensitivity	Use sunblockers	
	Teratogenic	Pregnancy contraindicated	
	Vesicant	Venospasm initially, use 2–8 mL sodium thiosulfate subcutaneously	

Dactinomycin (Actinomycin D, COSMEGEN)

Please tell the nurse or doctor if you have any of the following:

1. Poor appetite
2. Burning or redness at IV needle site
3. Diarrhea
4. Fatigue
5. Flu-like symptoms
6. Hair thinning
7. Mouth sores or white patches on the tongue
8. Nausea or vomiting
9. Pain or swelling at IV needle site
10. Skin color changes
11. Skin rash

Dactinomycin

DACTINOMYCIN   (Actinomycin D, Cosmegen)
Potentiates radiation toxicity.

Drug Action	Side Effects	Special Considerations	Cancers Effective Against
Antibiotic with inhibitory effect on bacteria and fungi as well as cytotoxic to nucleated cells. Cell cycle specific for G1 and S phases	Acniform rash	Occasional	Choriocarcinoma; Ewing's sarcoma; rhabdomyosarcoma; sarcoma botryoides; testicular; Wilms' tumor
	Alopecia.	Mild	
	Anorexia	Prolonged/common	
	Diarrhea.	Occasional	
	Erythema	Occasional	
	Flu-like syndrome	Occasional	
	GI effects	Dose limiting	
Nadir = 7 – 14 days	Hyperpigmentation	Occasional	
	Myelosuppression	Severe	
	Nausea/vomiting.	Moderate/severe in 2 – 5 hr, may last 2 days	
	Stomatitis.	Dose limiting	
	Vesicant.	2 – 8 mL sodium thiosulfate subcutaneously	

Daunorubicin Hydrochloride (Daunomycin, Rubidomycin, CERUBIDINE)

Please tell the nurse or doctor if you have any of the following:

1. Burning or redness at IV needle site
2. Diarrhea
3. Fatigue
4. Fever
5. Hair loss
6. Hives
7. Mouth sores
8. Nausea or vomiting
9. Pain or swelling at the IV needle site
10. Skin rash
11. Red urine

Daunorubicin Hydrochloride

DAUNORUBICIN HYDROCHLORIDE (Daunomycin, Rubidomycin, CERUBIDINE)
Incompatible with heparin.

Drug Action	Side Effects	Special Considerations	Cancers Effective Against
Antibiotic that inhibits synthesis of nucleic acids. Rapid effect on DNA Nadir = 10–14 days	Allergic reaction	Rare	Acute granulocytic leukemia (AGL); acute lymphocytic leukemia (ALL); acute myelogenous leukemia (AML); acute nonlymphocytic leukemia (ANLL); lymphoma; myeloma
	Alopecia	Common	
	Cardiotoxicity	Dose limiting	
	Diarrhea	Rare	
	Fever	Occasional	
	Malaise	Mild	
	Myelosuppression	Moderate at 60 mg/m^2; severe at 80 mg/m^2	
	Nausea/vomiting	Moderate/severe	
	Skin rash	Occasional	
	Stomatitis	Occasional	
	Thrombophlebitis	Rare	
	Urine is red	Common	
	Vesicant	Hydrocortisone cream applied topically or Solu-Cortef intradermally	

Dexamethasone (DECADRON)

Please tell the nurse or doctor if you have any of the following:

1. Depression
2. Excessive thirst
3. Menstrual changes
4. Mood changes
5. Muscle weakness
6. Nausea or vomiting
7. Nightmares
8. Skin color changes
9. Sweating more than usual
10. Swelling of face, hands, feet, or body trunk
11. Urination with greater frequency and/or volume

Dexamethasone

DEXAMETHASONE (DECADRON)
Contraindicated in systemic fungal infections.

Drug Action	Side Effects	Special Considerations	Cancers Effective Against
Synthetic adrenocortical steroid with potent anti-inflammatory effects. Modifies the body's immune responses and masks signs of infection	Diabetes mellitus	Enhances	Leukemia; lymphoma
	Edema	Common, dose dependent	
	Erythema	Occasional	
	GI toxicity	Increases with higher dosages	
	Menstrual irregularities	Occasional	
	Muscle weakness	Prolonged use	
	Psychic derangement	Mild	
	Sweating	Increased	

Diethylstilbestrol (DES, Estrostilben, Stibilium, Stilbestrol)

Please tell the nurse or doctor if you have any of the following:

1. Breast enlargement
2. Breathing difficulty
3. Chest pain
4. Confusion
5. Headache
6. Nausea or vomiting
7. Skin color yellow
8. Swelling of hands, feet, face, or trunk
9. Urination with greater frequency and/or volume
10. Vaginal bleeding

Diethylstilbestrol

DIETHYLSTILBESTROL (DES, Estrostilben, Stibilium, Stilbestrol)

Drug Action	Side Effects	Special Considerations	Cancers Effective Against
Synthetic estrogen that interferes with protein synthesis and alters cell metabolism by changing hormonal environments around the cell. Exact mechanism of action is not known	CHF	Rare	Breast; prostate
	Gynecomastia	Dose related	
	Hypercalcemia	Increased with bone metastasis or breast cancer	
	Hypertension	Occasional	
	Jaundice	Rare	
	Nausea/vomiting	Mild	
	Thrombosis	Rare	
	Urinary cystitis	Rare	
	Urinary frequency	Rare	
	Uterine bleeding	Occasional	

Doxorubicin Hydrochloride (ADM, ADRIAMYCIN)

Please tell the nurse or doctor if you have any of the following:

1. Chest pain
2. Face swelling
3. Fever
4. Hair loss
5. Hives
6. Mouth sores
7. Nails or knuckles change in color
8. Nausea or vomiting
9. Pain or swelling at the IV needle site

 Doxorubicin Hydrochloride

DOXORUBICIN HYDROCHLORIDE   (ADM, ADRIAMYCIN)

Incompatible with 5-FU or heparin. Do NOT administer in arm on same side as mastectomy.

Drug Action	Side Effects	Special Considerations	Cancers Effective Against
Antibiotic, cell cycle–nonspecific agent that is most active during DNA synthesis. Binds directly with DNA to inhibit synthesis Nadir = 10–14 days	Alopecia	Complete in 3–4 weeks	Bladder; breast; bronchogenic; gastric; germ cell; gynecologic; head and neck; hepatocellular; Hodgkin's disease; leukemia; lung; lymphoma; mesothelioma; multiple myeloma; mycosis fungoides; neuroblastoma; pancreas; prostate; renal; sarcoma; thyroid; Wilms' tumor
	Anaphylaxis	Rare	
	Bone marrow depression	Severe in 7 days; recovery 28 days	
	Cardiotoxicity	Dose limiting, permanent	
	Nausea/vomiting	Moderate/severe	
	Red urine	1–2 days after drug given	
	Skin reaction	Vein streaking, nail and knuckle hyperpigmentation, recall reaction to radiation sites, facial flushing with rapid infusion, sun sensitivity, use sunscreens	
	Stomatitis	Moderate	
	Vesicant	Stop infusion, apply cold compresses	

Estramustine Phosphate Sodium (Estradiol Mustard, ESTRACYT, EMCYT)

Please tell the nurse or doctor if you have any of the following:

1. Breast enlargement
2. Breathing difficulty
3. Chest pain
4. Nausea or vomiting

ESTRAMUSTINE PHOSPHATE SODIUM   (Estradiol Mustard, ESTRACYT, EMCYT)

Drug Action	Side Effects	Special Considerations	Cancers Effective Against
Elevates plasma concentrations of estradiol, producing estrogenic effects	Dyspnea. . . . . Occasional Edema . . . . Occasional Glucose tolerance . . . . . . Decreased Gynecomastia . . . . Common Hepatic dysfunction . . . . Increased LDH and SGOT common Myocardial infarction. . . . Increased risk Nausea. . . . . Mild Thrombosis . . . . Increased risk		Prostate

Estrogens, Conjugated (ESTRACON, PREMARIN)

Please tell the nurse or doctor if you have any of the following:

1. Acne
2. Appetite increased
3. Breast enlargement
4. Breathing difficulty
5. Chest pain
6. Diarrhea
7. Dizziness
8. Headache
9. Impotence
10. Menstrual period changes
11. Nausea
12. Skin color turns yellow
13. Vision changes of any kind

Estrogens, Conjugated

ESTROGENS, CONJUGATED   (ESTRACON, PREMARIN)

Drug Action	Side Effects	Special Considerations	Cancers Effective Against
Conjugated estrogen that increases DNA, RNA, and protein synthesis, reduces FSH and LH release from the pituitary, and helps in the development and maintenance of the female reproductive system and secondary sex characteristics	Acne	Occasional	Breast; prostate
	Amenorrhea	Occasional	
	Appetite increase	Occasional	
	Diarrhea	Rare	
	Dizziness	Rare	
	Dysmenorrhea	Occasional	
	Gynecomastia	Dose dependent	
	Headache	Occasional	
	Hypercalcemia	Rare	
	Hyperglycemia	Occasional	
	Impotence	Dose dependent	
	Jaundice	Rare	
	Nausea	Occasional	
	Shortness of breath	Rare	
	Thromboembolism	Rare	
	Visual disturbances	Rare	

Etoposide (VP-16, VP-16-213, VePesid)

Please tell the nurse or doctor if you have any of the following:

1. Poor appetite
2. Breathing difficulty
3. Chest pain
4. Chills
5. Diarrhea
6. Dizziness
7. Face swollen
8. Fever
9. Headache
10. Hives
11. Mouth sores
12. Nausea or vomiting
13. Numbness or tingling in hands or feet
14. Pain or swelling at IV needle site

Etoposide

ETOPOSIDE   (VP-16, VP-16-213, VePesid)
Unstable in D5W, may precipitate in NS within 30 minutes.

Drug Action	Side Effects	Special Considerations	Cancers Effective Against
Plant alkaloid, cell cycle-specific that inhibits DNA synthesis in S and G-2 stages Nadir = 7-10 days	Alopecia	Mild	Breast; bronchogenic; Hodgkin's disease; Kaposi's sarcoma; leukemia; lung; lymphoma; testicular
	Anaphylaxis	High risk	
	Anorexia	Mild	
	Bone marrow depression	Recovery in 20 days	
	Bronchospasm	Occasional	
	Diarrhea	Infrequent	
	Fever/chills	Mild	
	Headache	Moderate	
	Hypotension	Can be severe, keep recumbent	
	Nausea/vomiting	Mild	
	Peripheral neuropathy	Ataxia, foot drop, paresthesia	
	Stomatitis	Rare	
	Substernal pain	Occasional	
	Vesicant	1-6 mL Wydase subcutaneously followed by moderate heat	

Floxuridine (5-Fluorouracil Deoxyribonucleoside, 5-Fluorodeoxyuridine, FUDR)

Please tell the nurse or doctor if you have any of the following:

1. Diarrhea
2. Fatigue
3. Mouth sores
4. Nausea or vomiting
5. Skin dryness

Floxuridine   (5-Fluorouracil Deoxyribonucleoside, 5-Fluorodeoxyuridine, FUDR)

Drug Action	Side Effects	Special Considerations	Cancers Effective Against
Antimetabolite that interferes with the synthesis of DNA and RNA Nadir = 7–10 days	Abdominal cramps. . . . . . Occasional Biliary sclerosis . . . . Discontinue drug STAT Diarrhea. . . . . Common GI bleeding . . . . Occasional Keratitis . . . . Common Myelosuppression . . . . . . Mild Nausea/vomiting. . . . . . . Common Stomatitis. . . . . Common	Gastrointestinal, with metastasis to liver, gallbladder, and/or bile ducts; liver, primary or metastatic

5-Fluorouracil (5-FU, Adrucil, Efudex Topical)

Please tell the nurse or doctor if you have any of the following:

1. Poor appetite
2. Diarrhea
3. Eye sensitivity to light
4. Fever
5. Hair loss or thinning
6. Mouth sores
7. Muscle control problems
8. Nausea or vomiting
9. Nails brittle or easily breakable
10. Pregnancy or possible pregnancy
11. Skin dryness

5-Fluorouracil

5-FLUOROURACIL   (5-FU, ADRUCIL, EFUDEX TOPICAL)

Drug Action	Side Effects	Special Considerations	Cancers Effective Against
Antimetabolite cell cycle–specific agent that blocks the synthesis of nucleic acids necessary for the synthesis of DNA and RNA. S phase–specific Nadir = 7–14 days	Alopecia	Diffuse thinning	Bladder; bowel; breast; colon; gastric; head and neck; hepatocellular; lung; ovarian; pancreas; rectum; skin, basal cell; stomach
	Anorexia	Moderate	
	Bone marrow depression	Dose related	
	Diarrhea	May be severe	
	Hyperpigmentation	Veins darken, nails darken and crack	
	Nausea/vomiting	Precedes serious myelotoxicity. Dose dependent	
	Neurotoxicity	Cerebral ataxia	
	Photosensitivity	Use sunblockers	
	Pregnancy	Adverse effects on fetal development	
	Radiation recall	Use sunblockers	
	Skin dryness	Scaly dermatitis	
	Stomatitis	Preceded by sore mouth and tongue	

Fluoxymesterone (HALOTESTIN)

Please tell the nurse or doctor if you have any of the following:

1. Breathing difficulty
2. Breast enlargement
3. Clitoral enlargement
4. Confusion
5. Deepening of voice in females
6. Eye whites yellow in color
7. Menstrual changes
8. Penile erection of increased frequency or duration
9. Skin color yellow
10. Swelling of feet, face, arms, or trunk

Fluoxymesterone

FLUOXYMESTERONE (HALOTESTIN)

Drug Action	Side Effects	Special Considerations	Cancers Effective Against
Androgenic hormone that inhibits the release of testosterone through feedback inhibition of pituitary luteinizing hormone	Amenorrhea	Common	Breast (female); orchiectomy procedure; pituitary tumor
	CHF	Occasional	
	Edema	Occasional	
	Gynecomastia	Mild	
	Hepatotoxicity	Occasional	
	Hypercalcemia	Occasional with breast cancer	
	Jaundice	Rare	
	Penile erection	Increased frequency and duration occasionally	
	Virilization	Usual with high doses	

Hexamethylmelamine (HXM, HMM, *Altretamine*)

Please tell the nurse or doctor if you have any of the following:

1. Diarrhea
2. Fatigue
3. Nausea or vomiting
4. Numbness or tingling in hands or feet
5. Skin rash
6. Sleeping difficulty

Hexamethylmelamine

HEXAMETHYLMELAMINE   (HXM, HMM, Altretamine)

Drug Action	Side Effects	Special Considerations	Cancers Effective Against
Investigational agent that may be an alkylating agent activated in the body and also inhibits incorporation of precursors into DNA and RNA by means of an antimetabolite pathway Nadir = 3–4 weeks	Abdominal cramps	Mild	Breast; lung; lymphoma; ovarian
	Alopecia	Rare	
	CNS depression	Rare	
	Diarrhea	Occasional	
	Hallucinations	Rare	
	Myelosuppression	Mild/moderate, decreased WBCs and platelets	
	Nausea/vomiting	Moderate/severe	
	Peripheral neuropathy	Exacerbated with vincristine sulfate (see p. 174)	
	Rash	Mild	
	Sleep disturbance	Rare	

Hydrocortisone Sodium Succinate (A-HYDRO CORT, SOLU-CORTEF, S-CORTILEAN)

Please tell the nurse or doctor if you have any of the following:

1. Acne
2. Chest pain
3. Depressed mood
4. Appetite increased
5. Muscle weakness
6. Nausea or vomiting
7. Skin with red spots or black and blue marks
8. Sleeping problems
9. Swelling of face, arms, legs, or trunk

HYDROCORTISONE SODIUM SUCCINATE (A-HYDRO CORT, SOLU-CORTEF, S-CORTILEAN)

Contraindicated in systemic fungal infections. Acetate form NOT for IV usage.

Drug Action	Side Effects	Special Considerations	Cancers Effective Against
Cortisone that stabilizes leukocyte lysosomal membranes, thereby decreasing inflammation, suppressing the immune system, masking the signs and symptoms of infection, and stimulating bone marrow	Acne .... Occasional Appetite increased ..... Common CHF................. Rare Depression .... High doses Euphoria .... Occasional GI distress .... Dose dependent Hyperglycemia .... Occasional Hypokalemia .... Rare Insomnia .... Occasional Muscle weakness....... Prolonged usage Petechiae............ Occasional Wound healing .... Delayed		Leukemia; lymphoma

Hydroxyurea (HYD, HU, HUR, Hydrea)

Please tell the nurse or doctor if you have any of the following:

1. Poor appetite
2. Diarrhea
3. Fatigue
4. Mouth sores
5. Nausea or vomiting
6. Numbness or tingling in hands or feet
7. Skin rash

HYDROXYUREA (HYD, HU, HUR, HYDREA)
Radiation increases toxicity.

Drug Action	Side Effects	Special Considerations	Cancers Effective Against
Inhibition of S phase of DNA synthesis without interfering with synthesis of RNA or protein Nadir = 1–17 days	Anemia Anorexia GI toxicity Hallucinations Myelosuppression Nausea/vomiting Neurotoxicity Rash Renal toxicity Seizures Stomatitis	Moderate Moderate With doses >70 mg/kg Rare Moderate Mild Increased by 5-FU Occasional Occasional Rare Mild	Chronic granulocytic leukemia (CGL); chronic myelogenous leukemia (CML); head and neck; lung; melanoma; ovarian

Ifosfamide (HOLOXAN, IFX, IFEX)

Please tell the nurse or doctor if you have any of the following:

1. Confusion at times
2. Fatigue
3. Hair thinning
4. Nausea or vomiting
5. Urine that looks bloody

IFOSFAMIDE   (HOLOXAN, IFX, IFEX)

Drug Action	Side Effects	Special Considerations	Cancers Effective Against
Cell cycle – nonspecific alkylating agents that interfere with DNA replication and transcription	Alopecia	Mild	Breast; lung; lymphoma; ovarian; sarcoma; testicular
	CNS toxicity	Rare	
	Confusion	With high doses	
	Cystitis	Hemorrhagic	
	Fatigue	With high doses	
	Hallucinations	Rare	
Nadir = 7 – 14 days	Myelosuppression	Mild	
	Nephrotoxicity	With high doses	
	Phlebitis	Chemical	

Interferon (IF)

Please tell the nurse or doctor if you have any of the following:

1. Black and blue marks on skin
2. Chills
3. Dizziness
4. Fatigue
5. Fever
6. Headache
7. Nausea or vomiting
8. Nosebleed
9. Skin that itches

Interferon

INTERFERON   (IF)

Drug Action	Side Effects	Special Considerations	Cancers Effective Against
Glycoprotein (alpha, beta, gamma). Responds to infections and has a direct antitumor activity by binding to a cell membrane receptor that stimulates the immune system Nadir = several hours	Anorexia . . . . Blood pressure. . . . . Bone marrow depression . . . . Fatigue. . . . . Fever/chills . . . . Flu symptoms . . . . Metabolic. . . . . Nausea/vomiting. . . . . . . Neurologic toxicity . . . . . Renal toxicity. . . . . Skin reactions	Mild Hyper/hypotension Leukopenia and thrombocytopenia are comon Common Common Common Hypocalcemia, hyperkalemia, azotemia, or proteinuria Mild in 50% More likely in aged Increased BUN and creatinine Local redness, pruritus	Bladder; Kaposi's sarcoma; leukemia; lymphoma; melanoma; multiple myeloma; ovarian; renal

Interleukin-2 (IL-2)

Please tell the nurse or doctor if you have any of the following:

1. Black and blue marks on skin
2. Breathing difficulty
3. Chills
4. Confusion
5. Diarrhea
6. Fatigue
7. Headache
8. Nausea or vomiting
9. Skin rash
10. Swelling of feet, arms, hands, or trunk

INTERLEUKIN-2 (IL-2)

May be given intravenously, subcutaneously, intraperitoneally, intrahepatically, intrathecally, perilesionally.

Drug Action	Side Effects	Special Considerations	Cancers Effective Against
Lymphokine produced by activated T cells in response to macrophage antigens. Increases proliferation of T cells, synthesis of other cytokines, production of B-lymphocytes, proliferation of lymphokine-activated killer (LAK) cells	Anemia	Dose related	Breast; colorectal; head and neck; Hodgkin's disease; lung; lymphoma; melanoma; ovarian; renal
	Capillary leak syndrome	Dose > 1,000,000 U/kg	
	Diarrhea	Dose related	
	Dyspnea	Dose related	
	Flu-like syndrome	Common 2–4 hr after therapy	
	Mental changes	Rare	
	Nausea/vomiting	Dose related	
	Pulmonary edema	Acute	
	Rash	Pruritus mild	
	Renal dysfunction	Cumulative effect	
	Thrombocytopenia	Dose related	

Leucovorin (Citrovorum Factor, Folinic Acid, WELLCOVORIN)

Please tell the nurse or doctor if you have any of the following:

1. Breathing difficulty
2. Hives
3. Nausea or vomiting
4. Skin rash

LEUCOVORIN   (Citrovorum Factor, Folinic Acid, WELLCOVORIN)
May counteract bone marrow toxicity from trimethoprim and sulfa drugs.

Drug Action	Side Effects	Special Considerations	Cancers Effective Against
Antidote to folic acid antagonist by entering the general body pool of reduced folates. Antimetabolite, cell cycle–specific	Allergic sensitization .... Enhances toxicity of 5-FU .... Nausea/vomiting.......	Rare Diarrhea, dehydration Common. If vomiting occurs before next dose is due, folinic acid should be given parenterally without delay	MTX (methotrexate chemotherapy agent) rescue

Leuprolide Acetate (LUPRON)

Please tell the nurse or doctor if you have any of the following:

1. Breast enlargement
2. Constipation
3. Dizziness
4. Flushed face
5. Headache
6. Numbness in the fingers or toes
7. Pain in bones
8. Pain in general
9. Skin rash
10. Urination that is painful

LEUPROLIDE ACETATE (LUPRON)

Drug Action	Side Effects	Special Considerations	Cancers Effective Against
Acts as potent inhibitor of gonadotropin secretion by decreasing LH and FSH	Bone pain	Occasional	Prostate
	Constipation	Rare	
	Dizziness	Rare	
	Dysuria	Occasional	
	Gynecomastia	Occasional	
	Headache	Rare	
	Hot flashes	Occasional	
	Nausea/vomiting	Rare	
	Pain, general	Occasional	
	Paresthesia	Rare	
	Peripheral edema	Occasional	
	Rash	Rare	
	Testicular atrophy	Rare	

Lomustine (CCNU, CeeNU)

Please tell the nurse or doctor if you have any of the following:

1. Poor appetite
2. Breathing difficulty
3. Diarrhea
4. Fatigue
5. Hair loss
6. Mouth sores
7. Nausea or vomiting

LOMUSTINE (CCCNU, CeeNU)

Drug Action	Side Effects	Special Considerations	Cancers Effective Against
Nitrosourea that alkylates DNA and RNA and inhibits enzymatic processes in proteins Nadir = 21–28 days	Alopecia	Mild	Brain; central nervous system metastasis; colon; gastric; hepatocellular; Hodgkin's disease; lung; lymphoma; melanoma; multiple myeloma; ovarian; pancreas; rectum; stomach
	Anorexia	Common, lasts several days	
	Diarrhea	Common	
	Hepatotoxicity	Rare	
	Myelosuppression	Severe, delayed cumulative	
	Nausea/vomiting	Moderate/severe in 2–6 hours	
	Pulmonary	Fibrosis with prolonged use	
	Renal toxicity	Prolonged use	
	Stomatitis	Mild	

Mechlorethamine Hydrochloride (HN$_2$, Nitrogen Mustard, MUSTARGEN)

Please tell the nurse or doctor if you have any of the following:

1. Poor appetite
2. Breathing difficulty
3. Burning or redness at IV needle site
4. Chest pain
5. Chills
6. Diarrhea
7. Fever
8. Hair loss
9. Hives
10. Nausea or vomiting
11. Pain or swelling at IV needle site
12. Skin rash
13. Taste malfunction: foods taste metallic
14. Vein changes color

MECHLORETHAMINE HYDROCHLORIDE (HN$_2$, Nitrogen Mustard, MUSTARGEN)

Drug Action	Side Effects	Special Considerations	Cancers Effective Against
Alkylating agent that inhibits rapidly proliferating cells by interfering in DNA replication and transcription	Alopecia.................. Occasional Amenorrhea.............. Occasional Anaphylaxis .... Rare Anorexia.................. Common for days Chills .... Common Diarrhea................. Severe Fever .... Common Hypersensitivity.......... Rare Metallic taste .... Common Nausea/vomiting.......... Severe, lasts 2–12 hours Phlebitis................. Common Rash.................... Occasional Sterility.................. Occasional Tinnitus .... Occasional Vein discolored .... Common Vesicant................. 2 to 4 mL of 4% sodium thiosulfate subcutaneously and 5 mL into vein. Cold compresses for next 6–12 hours	Chronic granulocytic leukemia (CGL); chronic lymphocytic leukemia (CLL); chronic myelogenous leukemia (CML); Hodgkin's disease; lung; malignant effusions; mycosis fungoides; non-Hodgkin's lymphoma; polycythemia vera; sarcoma

Medroxyprogesterone Acetate (AMEN, CURRETAB, DEPO-PROVERA, PROVERA)

Please tell the nurse or doctor if you have any of the following:

1. Chest pain
2. Dizziness
3. Menstrual period changes
4. Nausea or vomiting
5. Sex drive that is decreased
6. Skin turns yellow
7. Swelling of face, arms, legs, or trunk

Medroxyprogesterone Acetate

MEDROXYPROGESTERONE ACETATE (AMEN, CURRETAB, DEPO-PROVERA, PROVERA)
Contraindicated in breast cancer and thromboembolic disorders.

Drug Action	Side Effects	Special Considerations	Cancers Effective Against
Progesterone derivative that inhibits pituitary gonadotropin secretion, thereby suppressing ovulation	Abscess . . . . IM use only Amenorrhea. . . . . Occasional Cervical mucus . . . . Thickens Dizziness . . . . Rare Dysmenorrhea. . . . . Occasional Edema . . . . Occasional Hyperglycemia . . . . Occasional Jaundice. . . . . Rare Libido decreased. . . . . . . Occasional Pulmonary embolism. . . . Rare		Endometrial; renal

Megestrol Acetate (MEGACE)

Please tell the nurse or doctor if you have any of the following:

1. Breathing problems
2. Chest pain
3. Confusion
4. Hair loss
5. Nausea or vomiting
6. Numbness in thumb or fingers
7. Pain in the calf of the leg
8. Skin rash
9. Swelling of the hands, arms, feet, calves, or trunk
10. Weight gain of more than 2 pounds in any one day

Megestrol Acetate

MEGESTROL ACETATE (MEGACE)

Drug Action	Side Effects	Special Considerations	Cancers Effective Against
Progestational drug whose antineoplastic effect is unknown, but an antiluteinizing effect is proposed	Alopecia. . . . . Mild Carpal tunnel syndrome . . . . Rare Dyspnea. . . . . Rare Edema . . . . Occasional Hyperglycemia . . . . Rare Nausea/vomiting. . . . . . . Rare Pulmonary emboli . . . . . . Rare Skin rash . . . . Rare Thrombophlebitis . . . . . . Rare Weight gain . . . . Common		Breast; endometrial

Melphalan (L-PAM, L-Phenylalanine Mustard, L-Sarcolysin, ALKERAN)

Please tell the nurse or doctor if you have any of the following:

1. Bleeding from anywhere on the body
2. Breathing difficulty
3. Fatigue
4. Hives
5. Missed menstrual period
6. Nausea or vomiting
7. Possible pregnancy
8. Skin rash

Melphalan

MELPHALAN   (L-PAM, L-Phenylalanine Mustard, L-Sarcolysin, ALKERAN)

Drug Action	Side Effects	Special Considerations	Cancers Effective Against
Alkylating agent that is a derivative of nitrogen mustard that interferes with DNA replication and transcription Nadir = 7 days	Amenorrhea . . . . Moderate Myelosuppression . . . . . . Moderate Nausea/vomiting . . . . Moderate Nonlymphocytic leukemia . . . . Occasional Ovarian suppression . . . . Occasional Pulmonary fibrosis . . . . . . Rare Rash . . . . Mild Sperm suppression . . . . . Occasional Urticaria . . . . Mild		Breast; melanoma; chronic granulocytic leukemia (CGL); chronic lymphocytic leukemia (CLL); multiple myeloma; osteosarcoma; ovarian

6-Mercaptopurine (6-MP, PURINETHOL)

Please tell the nurse or doctor if you have any of the following:

1. Poor appetite
2. Breathing difficulty
3. Fatigue
4. Fever
5. Mouth sores
6. Nausea or vomiting
7. Skin rash

6-Mercaptopurine

6-MERCAPTOPURINE   (6-MP, PURINETHOL)
Allopurinol decreases 6-MP to 25% of original dose.

Drug Action	Side Effects	Special Considerations	Cancers Effective Against
Antimetabolite purine analogue that interferes with nucleic acid biosynthesis Nadir = 5 days to 6 weeks	Allergic reaction	Fever, rash, eosinophilia	Acute granulocytic leukemia (AGL); acute lymphocytic leukemia (ALL); acute myelogenous leukemia (AML); chronic granulocytic leukemia (CGL); chronic lymphocytic leukemia (CLL)
	Anorexia	Occasional	
	Crystalluria	High doses only	
	Fever	Occasional	
	Hepatotoxicity	Cholestatis. Occurs with high doses. Increased risk when used with doxorubicin	
	Myelosuppression......	Mild, can be delayed up to 6 weeks	
	Nausea/vomiting.......	Uncommon	
	Pulmonary...........	Toxicity with prolonged usage	
	Stomatitis............	Occurs with high doses	

Methotrexate (MTX, FOLEX, MEXATE)

Please tell the nurse or doctor if you have any of the following:

1. Breathing difficulty
2. Diarrhea
3. Fatigue
4. Hair loss
5. Menstrual period problems
6. Mouth sores
7. Nausea
8. Skin rash
9. Throat that is sore or painful
10. Urine that is bright yellow

Methotrexate

METHOTREXATE (MTX, FOLEX, MEXATE)

Leucovorin rescue is mandatory with high dose MTX. Patient should avoid taking vitamins that contain folic acid, sulfonamides, ASA, tetracycline, PABA, phenytoin, and chloral hydrate.

Drug Action	Side Effects	Special Considerations	Cancers Effective Against
Antimetabolite that competes for folate binding sites that interfere with DNA synthesis. Nadir = 10–14 days	Alopecia	Mild	Acute lymphocytic leukemia (ALL); acute myelogenous leukemia (AML); breast; cervical; choriocarcinoma; central nervous system metastasis; head and neck; Hodgkin's disease; lung; lymphoma; mycosis fungoides; ovarian; sarcoma; testicular
	Bone marrow depression	Rapid onset with prolonged effect	
	Diarrhea	Dose limiting	
	Hepatic	Rare, cirrhosis, and necrosis	
	Hyperuricemia	Use allopurinol	
	Nausea	Mild	
	Neurologic	Usual with intrathecal mode	
	Pharyngitis	May be severe	
	Pulmonary	Toxicity with prolonged use	
	Renal	Failure in high doses	
	Reproductive	Menstrual problems, infertility, congenital malformation	
	Skin	Rash, brown color, photosensitivity	
	Stomatitis	May be severe	
	Urine	Colored bright yellow	

Methotrexate

Methylprednisolone Sodium Succinate (A-METHAPRED, Solu-Medrol)

Please tell the nurse or doctor if you have any of the following:

1. Acne
2. Chest pain
3. Depressed mood
4. Eating increased; appetite increased
5. Muscle weakness
6. Nausea or vomiting
7. Skin with red spots or black and blue marks
8. Sleeping problems
9. Swelling of face, arms, legs, or trunk

METHYLPREDNISOLONE SODIUM SUCCINATE (A-METHAPRED, SOLU-MEDROL)

Contraindicated in systemic fungal infections. Acetate form NOT for IV usage.

Drug Action	Side Effects	Special Considerations	Cancers Effective Against
Cortisone that stabilizes leukocyte lysosomal membranes, thereby decreasing inflammation, suppressing the immune system, masking the signs and symptoms of infection, and stimulating bone marrow	Acne	Occasional	Leukemia; lymphoma
	Appetite increased	Common	
	CHF	Rare	
	Depression	High doses	
	Euphoria	Occasional	
	GI distress	Dose dependent	
	Hyperglycemia	Occasional	
	Hypokalemia	Rare	
	Insomnia	Occasional	
	Muscle weakness	Prolonged usage	
	Petechiae	Occasional	
	Wound healing	Delayed	

Mitomycin C (MMC, MUTAMYCIN)

Please tell the nurse or doctor if you have any of the following:

1. Poor appetite
2. Breathing difficulty
3. Burning or redness at IV needle site
4. Diarrhea
5. Fatigue
6. Fever
7. Hair loss
8. Mouth sores
9. Nausea or vomiting
10. Pain in mouth or throat
11. Pain or swelling at IV needle site
12. Urination that is painful

Mitomycin C

MITOMYCIN C   (MMC, Mutamycin)

Drug Action	Side Effects	Special Considerations	Cancers Effective Against
Antibiotic that inhibitts DNA synthesis and RNA and protein at high doses Nadir = 21–28 days	Alopecia.	Rare	Bladder; breast; colon; head and neck; hepatoma; lymphoma; melanoma; multiple myeloma; pancreas; rectum; stomach
	Anorexia.	Common	
	Diarrhea.	Occasional	
	Dysuria.	Common with bladder instillation	
	Fever	Common	
	Hemolytic uremic syndrome	Rare	
	Mucositis	Occasional	
	Myelosuppression	Severe, especially platelets	
	Nausea/vomiting.	Moderate for 2–3 days	
	Phlebitis.	Chemically induced	
	Pulmonary	Fibrosis is rare	
	Stomatitis.	Occasional	
	Vesicant.	2–8 mL sodium thiosulfate subcutaneously followed by hydrocortisone topically	

Mitotane (*o,p'*-DDD, LYSODREN)

Please tell the nurse or doctor if you have any of the following:

1. Poor appetite
2. Dizziness
3. Eye sensitivity to light
4. Fatigue
5. Nausea or vomiting
6. Nosebleed
7. Numbness or tingling in hands or feet
8. Skin dryness
9. Skin rash

Mitotane

MITOTANE (*o,p'*-DDD, LYSODREN)
Interacts with CNS depressants, barbiturates, and warfarin.

Drug Action	Side Effects	Special Considerations	Cancers Effective Against
Modifies peripheral metabolism of steroids. Directly suppresses adrenal cortex	Adrenal suppression	Common	Adrenal carcinoma
	Anorexia	Common	
	CNS depression.	Common	
	Dermatitis	Common	
	Fatigue.	Common	
Nadir = 14–28 days	Hemorrhage	Rare	
	Hypothyroidism.	Occasional	
	Nausea/vomiting.	Severe	
	Neurotoxicity.	Rare	
	Orthostatic hypotension	Occasional	
	Visual disturbances	Sun sensitivity	

Mitoxantrone Hydrochloride (Alkylaminoanthraquinolone, DHAD, NOVANTRONE)

Please tell the nurse or doctor if you have any of the following:

1. Chest pain
2. Diarrhea
3. Fatigue
4. Fever
5. Hair loss
6. Mouth sores
7. Nausea or vomiting
8. Urine that is blue-green
9. Vein changes color

Mitoxantrone Hydrochloride

MITOXANTRONE HYDROCHLORIDE (Alkylaminoanthraquinolone, DHAD, NOVANTRONE)

Do not mix with heparin at all or with hydrocortisone phosphate in a plastic container.

Drug Action	Side Effects		Special Considerations	Cancers Effective Against
Cell cycle–nonspecific antibiotic that binds with DNA to inhibit synthesis of DNA and RNA	Alopecia	Mild		Acute granulocytic leukemia (AGL); acute nonlymphocytic leukemia (ANLL); breast; lymphoma
	Cardiotoxicity	Occasional in doxorubicin-treated persons		
	Diarrhea	Mild		
	Fatigue	Mild		
Nadir = 9–14 days	Fever	Rare		
	Myelosuppression	Mild, platelet sparing		
	Nausea/vomiting	Mild		
	Stomatitis	Mild		
	Urine discoloration	Blue-green		
	Vein discoloration	Blue-green		

Monoclonal Antibodies

Please tell the nurse or doctor if you have any of the following:

1. Breathing difficulty
2. Chills
3. Diarrhea
4. Fatigue
5. Fever
6. Flu-like syndrome
7. Hives
8. Nausea or vomiting
9. Skin redness

MONOCLONAL ANTIBODIES
Short IV infusion of 30 minutes to 2 hours.

Drug Action	Side Effects	Special Considerations	Cancers Effective Against
A hybridoma of specific B-cells fused with malignant B-cells or myeloma cells that results in a substance capable of producing large quantities of a specific antibody	Anaphylaxis . . . . Rare Diarrhea. . . . . Rare Erythema . . . . Generalized Flu-like symptoms . . . . . . Common, onset 2 – 8 hours after therapy Nausea/vomiting. . . . . . . Mild		Bladder; breast; colorectal; leukemia; lymphoma; ovarian; prostate; renal

Plicamycin (Mithramycin, MITHRACIN)

Please tell the nurse or doctor if you have any of the following:

1. Acne-like skin
2. Black and blue marks on skin
3. Burning or redness at IV needle site
4. Chills
5. Diarrhea
6. Fatigue
7. Fever
8. Headache
9. Mouth sores
10. Nausea or vomiting
11. Nosebleed

Plicamycin

PLICAMYCIN   (Mithramycin, MITHRACIN)

Drug Action	Side Effects	Special Considerations	Cancers Effective Against
Antibiotic that binds with DNA and inhibits DNA and RNA synthesis. Blocks hypercalcemic action of vitamin D	Bone marrow depression	Nadir of 2 weeks	Hypercalcemia of any disease or metastasis; testicular
	Diarrhea	Mild	
	Electrolyte imbalance	Low phosphorus, calcium, potassium	
	Epistaxis	Moderate, obtain prothrombin time	
Nadir = 7–14 days	Fever/chills	Mild	
	Headache	Severe	
	Hepatotoxicity	Liver necrosis possible	
	Iron deficiency	Mild	
	Nausea/vomiting	Moderate/severe. May last 12–14 hours	
	Neurotoxicity	Increased neuroexcitability	
	Renal toxic	Increased BUN/creatinine	
	Skin changes	Acne-like	
	Thrombocytopenia	Moderate/severe, common	
	Vesicant	1–2 mL DMSO subcutaneously followed by moderate heat	

Prednisone (Deltacortisone, Colisone, Deltasone, Meticorten, Orasone, Wojtab)

Please tell the nurse or doctor if you have any of the following:

1. No appetite
2. Breathing difficulty
3. Dizziness
4. Fatigue
5. Fever
6. Hair growth, new
7. Joint pain
8. Mood changes
9. Muscle weakness
10. Nausea
11. Swelling of face, arms, legs, or trunk

Prednisone

PREDNISONE   (Deltacortisone, COLISONE, DELTASONE, METICORTEN, ORASONE, WOJTAB)
Contraindicated in systemic fungal infections and in persons recently vaccinated especially for smallpox.

Drug Action	Side Effects	Special Considerations	Cancers Effective Against
Glucocorticoid that stabilizes leukocyte lysosomal membranes. Decreases inflammation, suppresses immune response, masks the signs and symptoms of infection, and stimulates bone marrow	Adrenal insufficiency .... Rare CHF .... Rare Delayed wound healing .... Dose dependent Edema .... Common, dose dependent Euphoria .... Dose dependent GI irritation .... Occasional Hirsutism .... Dose dependent Hyperglycemia .... Rare Hypocalcemia .... Rare Mood changes......... Occasional Muscle weakness....... High doses		Breast; Hodgkin's disease; leukemia; lymphoma; mycosis fungoides

Procarbazine Hydrochloride (MATULANE)

Please tell the nurse or doctor if you have any of the following:

1. Depressed mood
2. Fatigue
3. Flu-like symptoms
4. Nausea or vomiting
5. Nightmares
6. Numbness or tingling in hands or feet
7. Skin that is itchy, red, or peeling

PROCARBAZINE HYDROCHLORIDE (MATULANE)

Avoid concurrent use of MAOs, CNS depressants, ethanol, tricyclic antidepressants, and sympathomimetics.

Drug Action	Side Effects	Special Considerations	Cancers Effective Against
Cell cycle–nonspecific agent that inhibits DNA, RNA, and protein synthesis Nadir = 14–28 days	CNS depression	Caused by barbiturates, phenothiazines, antihistamines	Brain; CNS metastasis; Hodgkin's disease; liver; lung; lymphoma; melanoma; multiple myeloma; solid tumors
	Depression.	Rare	
	Dermatitis	Rare	
	Flu-like syndrome	Common	
	Hypertensive crisis	Caused by sympathomimetics, tricyclics, MAOs, foods high in tyramine (cheese, yogurt, soy sauce, bananas, raisins)	
	Myelosuppression	Moderate	
	Nausea/vomiting.	Moderate/severe	
	Neurotoxicity.	Rare	
	Nightmares	Rare	
	Pruritus.	Rare	

Semustine (Methyl CCNU)

Please tell the nurse or doctor if you have any of the following:

1. Loss of appetite
2. Bleeding anywhere from the body
3. Breathing difficulty
4. Fatigue
5. Nausea or vomiting
6. Pain on sides of hips or in the back

SEMUSTINE (Methyl CCNU)

Drug Action	Side Effects	Special Considerations	Cancers Effective Against
Nitrosourea that inhibits DNA cross-linked and enzymatic processes Nadir = 4-6 weeks	Anorexia . . . . Hepatic toxicity . . . . Myelosuppression. . . . . . Nausea/vomiting. . . . . . . Pulmonary fibrosis . . . . . . Renal toxicity	Common Occasional Common Acute, 2-6 hr Prolonged use Occasional	Brain; Hodgkin's disease; lymphoma

Streptozotocin (Streptozocin, STZ, ZANOSAR)

Please tell the nurse or doctor if you have any of the following:

1. Burning or redness at IV needle site
2. Chills
3. Diarrhea
4. Dizziness
5. Fatigue
6. Fever
7. Nausea or vomiting
8. Pain or swelling at IV needle site

STREPTOZOTOCIN   (Streptozocin, STZ, ZANOSAR)

Drug Action	Side Effects	Special Considerations	Cancers Effective Against
Nitrosourea that interferes with DNA, RNA, and protein replication. Crosses the blood-brain barrier Nadir = 7–14 days	Anemia	Mild	Carcinoid; colon; Hodgkin's disease; islet cell and malignant insulinoma; pancreas; stomach
	Chills	Rare	
	Diarrhea	Occasional	
	Eosinophilia	Mild	
	Extravasation	Pain, irritation, phlebitis	
	Fever	Rare	
	Hepatotoxicity	Transient, mild	
	Hyperinsulinemia	Occasional	
	Hypoglycemia	Secondary to insulin release	
	Myelosuppression	Mild, delayed	
	Nausea/vomiting	Severe in 1–4 hours	
	Nephrotoxicity	Glucosuria, proteinuria	
	Vesicant	Topical hydrocortisone cream	

Tamoxifen Citrate (NOLVADEX)

Please tell the nurse or doctor if you have any of the following:

1. Black and blue marks on skin
2. Double vision
3. Flushed face
4. Menstrual period problems
5. Nausea or vomiting
6. Nosebleed
7. Pain in bones
8. Skin rash

TAMOXIFEN CITRATE (NOLVADEX)

Drug Action	Side Effects	Special Considerations	Cancers Effective Against
Competitive inhibitor for estrogen receptors	Edema	Peripheral, rare	Breast; endometrium; hepatoma
	Hot flashes	Occasional	
	Hypercalcemia	Rare	
	Menstrual irregularity	Occasional	
	Nausea/vomiting	Occasional	
	Ocular changes	Rare	
	Pain	Existing soft tissue/bony lesions	
	Rash	Rare	
	Thrombocytopenia	Occasional	
	Vaginal bleeding/discharge	Rare	
	Weight gain	Occasional	

Teniposide (VM-26, VUMON)

Please tell the nurse or doctor if you have any of the following:

1. Breathing difficulty
2. Diarrhea
3. Dizziness
4. Fever
5. Hair loss
6. Nausea or vomiting
7. Pain or swelling at the IV needle site

Teniposide

TENIPOSIDE   (VM-26, VUMON)

Drug Action	Side Effects	Special Considerations	Cancers Effective Against
Plant alkaloid that causes permanent interruption in DNA replication prior to mitosis and inhibits the cell cycle	Alopecia................ Mild		Acute lymphocytic leukemia (ALL); bladder; brain; breast; chronic granulocytic leukemia (CGL); chronic lymphocytic leukemia (CLL); chronic myelogenous leukemia (CML); central nervous system metastasis; germ cell; Hodgkin's disease; leukemia; lung; lymphoma; melanoma; neuroblastoma; renal; solid tumors; testicular
	Anaphylaxis .... Rare, accompanied by cardiovascular collapse. Administering drug too fast increases risk of anaphylaxis		
	Bone marrow depression ... Mild, platelet sparing		
	Bronchospasm............ Occasional		
	Diarrhea................ Moderate		
	Fever .... Common		
	Hypotension .... Moderate		
	Nausea/vomiting......... Mild		
	Radiation recall .... Reactivates erythema at previous sites radiated		
	Stomatitis............... Rare		
	Vesicant................ Thrombophlebitis, apply warm compresses		

Testosterone (HISTERONE, MALOGEN, TESTOJECT)

Please tell the nurse or doctor if you have any of the following:

1. Acne
2. Dizziness
3. Nausea or vomiting
4. Skin turns yellow
5. Vaginal itching or burning
6. Weight gain

Testosterone

TESTOSTERONE (Histerone, Malogen, Testoject)

Drug Action	Side Effects	Special Considerations	Cancers Effective Against
Stimulates androgenic target cells	Acne	Occasional in females	Breast (postmenopausal)
	Hypercalcemia	Rare	
	Hypoglycemia	Occasional	
	Jaundice	Rare	
	Nausea/vomiting	Rare	
	Vaginitis	Rare	
	Weight gain	Common in females	

Testosterone

Thioguanine (6-TG)

Please tell the nurse or doctor if you have any of the following:

1. Diarrhea
2. Fatigue
3. Mouth sores
4. Nausea or vomiting
5. Skin that is itchy, red, or peeling
6. Skin rash

Thioguanine

THIOGUANINE (6-TG)

Drug Action	Side Effects	Special Considerations	Cancers Effective Against
Antimetabolite, purine antagonist that blocks DNA synthesis Nadir = 28 days	Dermatitis	Rare	Acute granulocytic leukemia (AGL); acute lymphocytic leukemia (ALL); acute myelogenous leukemia (AML); chronic granulocytic leukemia (CGL); chronic myelogenous leukemia (CML)
	Diarrhea	Rare, reduce dose to decrease diarrhea	
	Hepatotoxicity	Cholestatic, occasional	
	Hyperuricemia	Occasional	
	Myelosuppression	Mild	
	Nausea/vomiting	Rare	
	Rash	Rare	
	Stomatitis	Rare, reduce dose to decrease stomatitis	

Thiotepa (TEPA, AZIRIDINE)

Please tell the nurse or doctor if you have any of the following:

1. Poor appetite
2. Breathing difficulty
3. Dizziness
4. Fatigue
5. Fever
6. Hives
7. Menstrual period missed
8. Nausea or vomiting
9. Skin itchy
10. Skin rash
11. Urination that is painful
12. Urine looks bloody

Thiotepa

THIOTEPA (TEPA, AZIRIDINE)
Avoid concurrent succinylcholine administration.

Drug Action	Side Effects	Special Considerations	Cancers Effective Against
Alkylating agent that releases ethylenimine radicals, which disrupt the bonds of DNA, particularly by alkylation of guanine at N-7 position Nadir = 14–21 days	Allergic reaction	Rare	Bladder; breast; central nervous system malignancy; Hodgkin's disease; lymphoma; lymphosarcoma; malignant effusions; ovarian
	Amenorrhea	Rare	
	Anorexia	Moderate	
	Cystitis	Only intrathecal	
	Dizziness	Occasional	
	Fever	Mild	
	Headache	Mild	
	Hives	Rare	
	Leukopenia	Occasional after bladder instillation	
	Myelosuppression	Moderate, potentiated by prior radiation and other alkylating agents	
	Nausea/vomiting	Mild with intracavitary instillation	
	Pruritus	Rare	
	Rash	Rare	
	Sterility	Ovary or sperm suppression	

Tumor Necrosis Factor (TNF, Cachectin)

Please tell the nurse or doctor if you have any of the following:

1. No appetite
2. Chills
3. Diarrhea
4. Dizziness
5. Fatigue
6. Fever
7. Headache
8. Nausea or vomiting
9. Pain

TUMOR NECROSIS FACTOR   (TNF, Cachectin)
May be given intravenously, intramuscularly, subcutaneously, or directly into the bladder.

Drug Action	Side Effects	Special Considerations	Cancers Effective Against
Macrophage secretion that binds to receptors on tumor cells and destroys the cells. Mechanism of action unknown	Anorexia	Common	Bladder; colon; hepatic; rectal
	Chills	Occasional	
	Diarrhea	Rare	
	Dizziness	Occasional	
	Flu-like syndrome	Common	
	Headache	Occasional	
	Hepatic dysfunction	Rare	
	Nausea/vomiting	Occasional	
	Orthostatic hypotension	Common	
	Pain at tumor site	Severe	

Vinblastine Sulfate (VLB, VELBAN)

Please tell the nurse or doctor if you have any of the following:

1. Confusion at times
2. Constipation
3. Depressed mood
4. Fever
5. Hair loss
6. Headache
7. Jaw pain
8. Mouth sores
9. Nausea or vomiting
10. Numbness or tingling in hands or feet
11. Pain or swelling at the IV needle site

Vinblastine Sulfate

VINBLASTINE SULFATE (VLB, Velban)

Leukocytes nadir in 5 to 9 days; recovery in 14 to 21 days.

Drug Action	Side Effects	Special Considerations	Cancers Effective Against
Plant alkaloid, phase-specific, arrests mitosis in metaphase by binding with microtubular proteins	Alopecia	Moderate	Breast; germ cell; head and neck; Hodgkin's disease; Kaposi's sarcoma; lymphoma; mycosis fungoides; testicular
	Bone marrow depression	Dose related	
	CNS toxicity	Confusion, depression	
	Constipation	May be a sign of paralytic ileus	
	Corneal ulcer	If eye splashed	
Nadir = 7 – 14 days	Cranial nerve toxicity	VI (abducens); VII (facial)	
	Headache	Moderate	
	Jaw pain	Moderate, dose limiting	
	Nausea/vomiting	Occasional	
	Neurotoxicity	At doses >20 mg	
	Ocular problem	Rare, diplopia	
	Peripheral neuropathy	Ataxia, foot drop, paresthesia	
	Reproductive	Possible teratogenic, aspermia	
	Stomatitis	Moderate	
	Vesicant	1 – 6 mL hyaluronidase subcutaneously, then warm compresses	

Vinblastine Sulfate

Vincristine Sulfate (VCR, ONCOVIN)

Please tell the nurse or doctor if you have any of the following:

1. Poor appetite
2. Confusion at times
3. Constipation
4. Depressed mood
5. Double vision
6. Hair loss
7. Jaw pain
8. Numbness or tingling in hands or feet
9. Pain or swelling at the IV needle site

Vincristine Sulfate

VINCRISTINE SULFATE (VCR, ONCOVIN)

Drug Action	Side Effects	Special Considerations	Cancers Effective Against
Plant alkaloid, cell cycle–specific, arrests mitosis at metaphase and inhibits cell division Nadir = 4–10 days	Alopecia	Mild	Acute lymphocytic leukemia (ALL); blast crisis; breast; bronchogenic; cervical; colorectal; head and neck; Hodgkin's disease; leukemia: acute granulocytic leukemia (AGL)/chronic lymphocytic leukemia (CLL); lung; lymphoma medulloblastoma; melanoma; multiple myeloma; mycosis fungoides; neuroblastoma; sarcoma; testicular; Wilms' tumor
	Anorexia	Mild	
	Bone marrow depression	Mild leukopenia	
	CNS toxicity	Confusion, depression	
	Constipation	Stool softener	
	GI symptoms	Rare	
	Hyponatremia	Occasional	
	Jaw pain	Moderate. Dose limiting	
	Neurologic	Temporary or permanent paresthesis, motor weakness, loss of deep tendon reflex, vocal cord paralysis	
	Ocular problems	Rare. Diplopia, photophobia	
	Reproductive	Impotence	
	SIADH	Occasional	
	Vesicant	1–6 mL Wydase subcutaneously followed by moderate heat	

Vindesine Sulfate (Desacetylvinblastine Amide, DAVA, VND, ELDISINE)

Please tell the nurse or doctor if you have any of the following:

1. Burning or redness at IV needle site
2. Constipation
3. Diarrhea
4. Fatigue
5. Jaw pain
6. Mouth sores
7. Nausea or vomiting
8. Numbness or tingling in hands or feet
9. Pain in mouth or throat
10. Pain or swelling at the IV needle site
11. Urination problems

VINDESINE SULFATE   (Desacetylvinblastine Amide, DAVA, VND, ELDISINE)
Decrease dose with increased bilirubin.

Drug Action	Side Effects	Special Considerations	Cancers Effective Against
Plant alkaloid and mitotic spindle inhibitor Nadir = 3–11 days	Constipation .... Rare Diarrhea................ Occasional Jaw pain................. Severe Mucositis .... Mild Myelosuppression .... Mild/moderate Nausea/vomiting......... Occasional Neurotoxicity............. Great cumulative potential with other vinca alkaloids Paralytic ileus............. Rare Phlebitis................. Rare Stomatitis .... Mild Urinary retention......... Rare Vesicant................. 1–6 mL Wydase subcutaneously followed by moderate heat		Acute granulocytic leukemia (AGL); acute lymphocytic leukemia (ALL); blast crisis in acute myelogenous leukemia (AML); breast; leukemia; lung lymphoma; melanoma

Habermann, T. M. Alpha interferon: Progress and perspectives in the biotherapy of chronic myelogenous leukemia. Oncology Nursing Forum (Suppl.) *16*(6):8–11, 1989.

Johnson, B. L., and Gross, J. Handbook of Oncology Nursing. New York: John Wiley & Sons, 1985.

Montrose, P. A. Extravasation management. Seminars in Oncology Nursing *3*(2):128–132, 1987.

National Institutes of Health, U.S. Department of Health and Human Services. Cancer Rates and Risks, 3rd. ed. NIH Publ. No. 85-691, Bethesda, MD, April 1985.

Oncology Nursing Society. Cancer Chemotherapy Guidelines, Module V, Recommendations for The Management of Extravasation and Anaphylaxis. Pittsburgh: Oncology Nursing Society, 1988.

Parkinson, D. R. The Role of Interleukin-2 in the Biotherapy of Cancer. Oncology Nursing Forum (Suppl.) *16*(6):16–20, 1989.

Tenenbaum, L. Cancer Chemotherapy: A Reference Guide. Philadelphia: W. B. Saunders Co., 1989.

Vadham-Raj, S. Clinical applications of colony-stimulating factors. Oncology Nursing Forum (Suppl.) *16*(6):20–26, 1989.

Yasko, J. M., and Dudjak, L. A. Biological Response Modifier Therapy: Symptom Management. Emeryville, CA: Cetus Corporation, Park Row Publishers, 1990.

Ziegfeld, C. Core Curriculum for Oncology Nursing. Philadelphia: W. B. Saunders Co., 1987.

Alternative Drug Name	See Chemotherapeutic Agent Card
Actinomycin D	Dactinomycin
ADM	Doxorubicin hydrochloride
Adriamycin	Doxorubicin hydrochloride
Adrucil	5-Fluorouracil
A-hydro Cort	Hydrocortisone sodium succinate
Alkeran	Melphalan
Alkylamino-anthraquinolone	Mitoxantrone hydrochloride
Altretamine	Hexamethylmelamine
Amen	Medroxyprogesterone acetate
A-methaPred	Methylprednisolone sodium succinate
Arabino-sylcytosine	Cytarabine
Ara-C	Cytarabine
Aziridine	Thiotepa
BCNU	Carmustine

Alternative Drug Name	See Chemotherapeutic Agent Card
BiCNU	Carmustine
Blenoxane	Bleomycin
Bleo	Bleomycin
BUS	Busulfan
Cachectin	Tumor necrosis factor
CCNU	Lomustine
CDDP	Cisplatin
CeeNU	Lomustine
Cerubidine	Daunorubicin hydrochloride
CHL	Chlorambucil
Citrovorum Factor	Leucovorin
CLB	Chlorambucil
Colisone	Prednisone
Cosmegen	Dactinomycin
CTX	Cyclophosphamide
Curretab	Medroxyprogesterone acetate
CYT	Cyclophosphamide

Alternative Drug Name	*See* Chemotherapeutic Agent Card	Alternative Drug Name	*See* Chemotherapeutic Agent Card
Cytosar	Cytarabine	DTIC-Dome	Dacarbazine
Cytoxan	Cyclophosphamide	Efudex	5-Fluorouracil
Daunomycin	Daunorubicin hydrochloride	Eldisine	Vindesine sulfate
DAVA	Vindesine sulfate	Elspar	L-Asparaginase
DDP	Cisplatin	Emcyt	Estramustine phosphate sodium
Decadron	Dexamethasone	Endoxana	Cyclophosphamide
Deltacortisone	Prednisone	Estracon	Estrogens, conjugated
Deltasone	Prednisone	Estracyt	Estramustine phosphate sodium
Depo-Provera	Medroxyprogesterone acetate	Estradiol mustard	Estramustine phosphate sodium
DES	Diethylstilbestrol	Estrostilben	Diethylstilbestrol
Desacetylvinblastine amide	Vindesine sulfate	5-Fluorodeoxy-uridine	Floxuridine
DHAD	Mitoxantrone hydrochloride	5-Fluorouracil Deoxyribo-nucleoside	Floxuridine
Diamminedichloro-platinum	Cisplatin		
DTIC	Dacarbazine		

Alternative Drug Name	See Chemotherapeutic Agent Card	Alternative Drug Name	See Chemotherapeutic Agent Card
Folex	Methotrexate	IFX	Ifosfamide
Folinic acid	Leucovorin	IL-2	Interleukin-2
5-FU	5-Fluorouracil	Imidazole carboxamide	Dacarbazine
FUDR	Floxuridine	L-ASP	L-Asparaginase
G-CSF	Colony-stimulating factor	Leukeran	Chlorambucil
GM-CSF	Colony-stimulating factor	L-PAM	Melphalan
Halotestin	Fluoxymesterone	L-Phenylalanine mustard	Melphalan
Histerone	Testosterone	L-Sarcolysin	Melphalan
HMM	Hexamethylmelamine	Lupron	Leuprolide acetate
HN_2	Mechlorethamine hydrochloride	Lysodren	Mitotane
Holoxan	Ifosfamide	Malogen	Testosterone
HU	Hydroxyurea	Matulane	Procarbazine hydrochloride
HUR	Hydroxyurea	M-CSF	Colony-stimulating factor
HXM	Hexamethylmelamine	Megace	Megestrol acetate
HYD	Hydroxyurea	Methyl CCNU	Semustine
Hydrea	Hydroxyurea	Meticorten	Prednisone
IF	Interferon		
IFEX	Ifosfamide		

Alternative Drug Name	See Chemotherapeutic Agent Card	Alternative Drug Name	See Chemotherapeutic Agent Card
Mexate	Methotrexate	Platinol	Cisplatin
Mithracin	Plicamycin	Premarin	Estrogens, conjugated
Mithramycin	Plicamycin	Procytox	Cyclophosphamide
MMC	Mitomycin C	Provera	Medroxyprogesterone acetate
6-MP	6-Mercaptopurine	Purinethol	6-Mercaptopurine
MTX	Methotrexate	Rubidomycin	Daunorubicin hydrochloride
Mustargen	Mechlorethamine hydrochloride	S-Cortilean	Hydrocortisone sodium succinate
Mutamycin	Mitomycin C	Solu-Cortef	Hydrocortisone sodium succinate
Myleran	Busulfan	Solu-Medrol	Methylprednisolone sodium succinate
Neosar	Cyclophosphamide	Stibilium	Diethylstilbestrol
Nitrogen mustard	Mechlorethamine hydrochloride	Stilbestrol	Diethylstilbestrol
Nolvadex	Tamoxifen citrate	Streptozocin	Streptozotocin
Novantrone	Mitoxantrone hydrochloride	STZ	Streptozotocin
Oncovin	Vincristine sulfate	TACE	Chlorotrianisene
o,p'-DDD	Mitotane		
Orasone	Prednisone		
Paraplatin	Carboplatin		

Alternative Drug Name	*See* Chemotherapeutic Agent Card	Alternative Drug Name	*See* Chemotherapeutic Agent Card
TEPA	Thiotepa	VM-26	Teniposide
Testoject	Testosterone	VND	Vindesine sulfate
6-TG	Thioguanine	VP-16	Etoposide
TNF	Tumor necrosis factor	VP-16-213	Etoposide
VCR	Vincristine sulfate	Vumon	Teniposide
Velban	Vinblastine sulfate	Wellcovorin	Leucovorin
VePesid	Etoposide	Wojtab	Prednisone
VLB	Vinblastine sulfate	Zanosar	Streptozotocin

ISBN 0-7216-3187-8